NOVEL IMPLICATIONS OF EXOSOMES IN DIAGNOSIS AND TREATMENT OF CANCER AND INFECTIOUS DISEASES

Edited by **Jin Wang**

Novel Implications of Exosomes in Diagnosis and Treatment of Cancer and Infectious Diseases
http://dx.doi.org/10.5772/65504
Edited by Jin Wang

Contributors

Sin-Yeang Teow, Suat-Cheng Peh, Mustafa Kotmakçı, Gülşah Erel Akbaba, Jin Wang, Lucia Paolini, Andrea Zendrini, Doris Ricotta, Paolo Bergese, Giuseppe Di Noto, Bárbara Adem, Sonia Melo, Muhammad Nawaz, Farah Fatima, Jeremy Squire, Duc Bach Nguyen, Thuy Ly Thi Bich, Ingolf Bernhardt, Gulfaraz Khan, Waqar Ahmed, Pretty Philip

Published by InTech
Janeza Trdine 9, 51000 Rijeka, Croatia

Publishing Process Manager Romina Rovan
Technical Editor SPi Global
Cover InTech Design team

First published July, 2017
Printed in Croatia
Legal deposit, Croatia: National and University Library in Zagreb

Additional hard copies can be obtained from orders@intechopen.com

Novel Implications of Exosomes in Diagnosis and Treatment of Cancer and Infectious Diseases, Edited by Jin Wang
p. cm.
Print ISBN 978-953-51-3335-3
Online ISBN 978-953-51-3336-0

Meet the editor

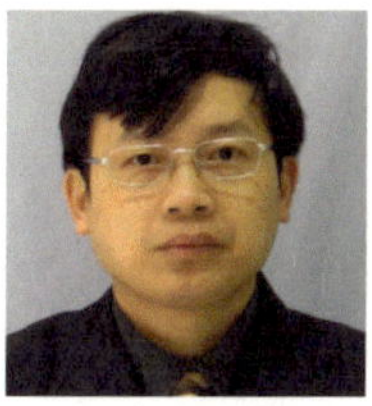

Professor Jin Wang is a PI at Shanghai Public Health Clinical Center, Fudan University, China. Dr. Wang has been working in the fields of cancer and infectious diseases. A major focus of his research is to develop novel early detection biomarkers of human cancers utilizing various state-of-the-art genomic technologies, and he has been able to identify several interesting candidate biomarkers of human pancreatic cancers and liver cancer. Dr. Wang has authored/coauthored 3 patents (*U.S. WO Patent WO/2012/030,956; P.R. China Patent NO: 99113481.8*) and over 30 SCI publications with a citation rate of over 1000. He has received the prestigious *Anne Eastland Spears Fellowship Award* in Gastrointestinal Cancer Research from the University of Texas, MD Anderson Cancer Center in the USA, and three independent fellowships from reputed institutions including NIH/NIDDK (USA). His laboratory conducts basic and translational research in the following areas: (1) development of novel early detection biomarkers of human gastrointestinal (GI) cancers and (2) pharmacologic *ascorbic acid, all-trans retinoid acid,* and *ncRNAs* for treatment of cancer and infectious diseases.

Contents

Preface

Exosome research is a young and rapidly changing field. It is exciting to write about it, but it is also hard to know when to stop, since new results appear at frequent intervals. This book provides a forum for novel implications of exosomes in diagnosis and treatment of cancer and infectious diseases. It is a timely reference to explore the early detection biomarkers of cancer and infectious diseases and will help develop successful therapeutic intervention in these diseases in the future.

For clarity, the eight chapters of this book have been clustered into three parts. Part I clusters Chapters 1–3, outlining the exosomes in cancer. The topics deal with the mechanisms of tumor formation under the exosomes' action, showing how circulating exosomes have come into the spotlight of research as a high potential biomarker of pancreatic cancer and multiple myeloma, and outlining the application of exosomes as transfer vector in tumor therapeutics. As a high potential source of "liquid biopsies," exosomes, which are secreted by fusing the intracellular multivesicular body with cell membrane, have relative stability and composition covering the whole range of cancer-related biomarkers including the cells' proteins, lipids, DNA, and RNA. The emphasis in the first part of the book is on exosomal lncRNAs and miRNAs, which can serve as diagnostic and prognostic factors, complementing clinical and pathological parameters in the effort to predict the outcome of patients with pancreatic cancer. Chapter 2 discusses that multiple myeloma and monoclonal gammopathy of undetermined significance (MGUS) exosomes are different in concentration, biological activity, and biochemical markers. These differences seem to be related to the free light chains associated to exosomes and their pro-pathogenic properties. Knowledge in the field of tumor-derived exosomes advanced so quickly, which lead to numerous findings correlating these extracellular vesicles with tumor growth, metastatic process, and their close association with the immune system. Chapter 3 presents animal models in exosome research, where Dr. Melo presents that genetically engineered mouse models can be a promising approach to address the current technical limitations allowing tracing tumor-derived exosomes while retaining the animal immune system.

Part II comprises two chapters focusing on exosomes in viral infection. Chapter 4 provides an overview of our current understanding of exosome biogenesis and how this normal physiological process is hijacked by some pathogenic viruses. The potential roles of exosomes in viral pathogenesis are also discussed in Chapter 4. Details relating to exosomes from Epstein-Barr virus (EBV)-associated cancers are included in Chapter 5. Current evidences support the pathogenic roles of exosomes in EBV-related cancers as biomarkers in cancer diagnostics and therapy response. Part II highlights the potential challenges in the development of exosome-based biomarkers for clinical application in infectious diseases.

The last three chapters in Part III explain the formation and release of extracellular vesicles (EVs), microvesicles (MVs), and exosomes. Exosomes are a class of EVs of small size (40–120 nm) originating in multivesicular endosomes and can be released from a wide range of cells, which differ in size from MVs (50–1000 nm) and apoptotic bodies (800–5000 nm) and are secreted directly from the cell membrane in budding form. Details of how to isolate exosomes from liquid biopsy and blood are given in Part III, where recent progress and remaining challenges in the isolation of EVs for diagnosis and treatment of cancer and infectious diseases are discussed.

This book is intended to provide deep coverage of topics that we feel are reasonably well understood. Rapid progress in the field of exosomes made it possible to reduce the coverage of less significant areas. The book is designed for different readers although it is hard to simultaneously cover all the areas of exosomes in this book. I believe that one should solve the basic exosome problem before starting to worry about implications of exosomes in diagnosis and treatment of cancer and infectious diseases.

Jin Wang PhD
Professor
Scientific Research Center
Shanghai Public Health Clinical Center
Fudan University

Section 1

Exosome in Cancer

Chapter 1

Novel Implications of Exosomes and lncRNAs in the Diagnosis and Treatment of Pancreatic Cancer

Jin Wang, Xuan Zhang, Chunxia Ji, Lei Zhang, Yang Di, Wenhui Lou, Xiaoyan Zhang and Jianqing Xu

Additional information is available at the end of the chapter

http://dx.doi.org/10.5772/intechopen.69510

Abstract

Pancreatic cancer remains a leading cause of cancer-related deaths. Most patients are present with advanced stages of the disease at the time of diagnosis; thus, surgery, which is the best curative option for this malignancy, is no longer an effective treatment modality for affected individuals. As a likely source of "liquid biopsies," exosomes, which are secreted by fusing intracellular multivesicular bodies with cell membranes, have relative stability and composition, allowing them to cover the entire range of cancer-related biomarkers, including cellular proteins, lipids, DNA, RNA, miRNA, and long non-coding RNAs (lncRNAs). To explore the early detection biomarkers of pancreatic cancer and to develop successful therapeutic intervention for this disease, assessing the implications of exosomes in pancreatic cancer patients is essential. In this chapter, we wish to focus on the possibility of using exosomes and lncRNAs in the clinical management of patients with pancreatic cancer. We will discuss the mechanisms of tumor formation under the exosomal action, demonstrate how circulating exosomes and lncRNAs have come into the research spotlight as likely biomarkers of pancreatic cancer, and discuss the applications of exosomes as transfer vectors in tumor therapeutics.

Keywords: exosomes, lncRNA, pancreatic cancer, biomarkers, diagnosis, therapeutic intervention

1. Introduction

1.1. Exosomes, ncRNAs, and lncRNAs

Exosomes are a class of small (40–120 nm) extracellular vesicles (EVs) that originate in multivesicular endosomes [1–3] and can be released from a wide range of cells, including cancer cells [4]. Exosomes differ in size from microvesicles (50–1000 nm) and apoptotic bodies (800–5000 nm) and are secreted directly from the cell membrane in a budding form [5–7]. Late endosomes released from multivesicular bodies (MVBs) are integrated with the cell membrane in the extracellular matrix during the release of exosomes. Exosomes released into the extracellular environment can be utilized by tumor cells to alter the tumor microenvironment or to provide a favorable microenvironment for distant metastases by affecting distant organs [8–10]. Therefore, exosomes serve as efficient vehicles for long- and short-distance intercellular communication by signaling molecules in the form of lipids, proteins, DNA, RNAs, and non-coding RNAs (ncRNAs) [11]. Exosomes play an important role in signal transduction between cells.

In the complicated human genome, approximately 2% of the genomic sequence encodes proteins involved in biological progression [12], of which approximately 90% are ncRNAs. ncRNAs are described as the "noise" of the genome in their primary form, and they can be divided into two subgroups: small ncRNAs (sncRNAs) and long ncRNAs (lncRNAs) [13–16]. If RNA is <200 nt in length, the ncRNAs are defined as sncRNAs, which includes microRNAs (also called miRNAs or miRs). Conversely, long non-coding RNAs (lncRNAs) are >200 nt in length. Previous studies have reported that lncRNAs are involved in numerous physiological and pathological processes.

In recent years, an increasing number of lncRNAs have been investigated, and play a vital role in various major biological processes associated with promoting proliferation, invasion, and migration metabolism [17–19]. Increasing evidence points to important functional or regulatory roles of lncRNAs in cellular processes, including the cell cycle, proliferation, apoptosis [20–22], RNA processing [23], chromatin modification [24, 25], genomic reprogramming [26, 27], and gene imprinting [28]. They also play a role in cancers resulting from aberrant lncRNA expression. Recent findings indicate that lncRNAs are dysregulated in many kinds of cancer, including pancreatic cancer (PaCa), and they are closely related with tumorigenesis, metastasis, prognosis, and diagnosis.

2. The physiological function of exosomes

Exosomes carry a variety of substances from secreted cells, including proteins, lipids, DNA, RNA, and ncRNA [29, 30]. The intercellular communication regulated by exosomes is not only involved in regulating the physiological processes of normal cells but also participates in many pathological processes associated with disease development, including tumors [31–33]. Exosomes regulate biological activity through the rapid reaction of signal molecules on their surface or by the release of extracellular biologically active substances. Exosomal biological activity is mainly determined by its components (i.e., the exosome cell source) [8–10]. Exosomes, which use autocrine, paracrine, and endocrine signaling to exchange biological information, are involved in the transmission of substances and signals between cells.

In addition, exosomes have immunomodulatory function [34]. Antigen-presenting cell (APC)-derived exosomes can promote the proliferation of T lymphocytes and induce antitumor immune responses in vivo. Exosomes have the features of their original cells because they bring DNA, RNA, and proteins from the original cell and carry a variety of proteins on their surface. Since exosomes are released from endosomes, they carry certain endosomal-specific proteins, including GTPases, flotillin, Alix, Tsg101, CD81 and CD82, heat shock proteins Hsp70 and Hsp90, and epithelial cell adhesion molecules [35–38] that are involved in exosome formation.

If exosomes are secreted by tumor cells, they can kill the tumor cells by providing information to cytotoxic T lymphocytes by cross-reacting with antigen-presenting cells [39]. However, exosomes from tumor cells have a dual role in that they have antitumor activity and also promote tumor growth. For example, exosomes from colorectal cancer cells contain cell cycle-related mRNAs that promote the proliferation of endothelial cells, which can induce tumor angiogenesis [40]. Exosomes obtained from gastric cancer cells promote tumor progression by activating the NF-kB pathway in macrophages [41]. In ovarian cancer, epithelial ovarian cancer (EOC) cell-derived exosomes promote ovarian cancer metastasis and deterioration by transferring CD44 to peritoneal cells [42].

3. Exosomes as novel biomarkers of cancer

The identification of cancer-specific exosomes in bodily fluids, such as serum, plasma, and urine, will be useful for the detection of cancer and will allow for the identification of specific DNA, RNA, and protein content in the absence of contamination from non-cancerous exosomes [43]. The proteoglycan glypican-1 (GPC1) is highly expressed in tumor cell-derived exosomes. GPC1 has been shown to be a specific, sensitive marker in serum from pancreatic patients that are in both the early and late stages but not in benign pancreatic diseases [43]. CD24 and EpCAM are tumor-derived exosome markers isolated by immune-affinity techniques involving anti-CD24 and anti-EpCAM magnetic beads [44]. In serum, CD24 and EpCAM serve as early diagnosis biomarkers [44], while fibronectin can serve as an early diagnosis biomarker in plasma. The ELISA method has been used to detect fibronectin [45]. The levels of exosomal EDIL3 from breast cancer patients can be dramatically reduced with surgery, indicating that EDIL3 can also serve as a diagnostic and prognostic biomarker [46]. Survivin expression has been shown to be significantly increased in patients with prostate cancer, but lower survivin expression has been found in benign prostatic hyperplasia (BPH) and healthy subjects. Additionally, the levels of survivin in BPH and healthy subjects are not significantly different. Thus, survivin can be used as a new diagnostic indicator of prostate cancer [47].

Separated and purified exosomes not only contain mRNA and miRNA but also tRNA and some lncRNA [11, 48–50]. Six miRNAs (miR-19b-3p, miR-21-5p, miR-221-3p, miR-409-3p, miR-425-5p, and miR-584-5p) were found to be upregulated in lung adenocarcinoma [51]. Eight miRNAs (miR-21, miR-141, miR-200a, miR-200c, miR-200b, miR-203, miR-205, and miR-214) have served as diagnostic biomarkers for ovarian cancer, and these miRNAs have also been identified in exosomes from ovarian cancer patients [52]. miRNAs can also be diagnostic biomarkers for esophageal squamous cell cancer (ESCC), as the serum levels of exosomal miR-21 from patients with ESCC are significantly higher than those of patients with benign diseases without systemic inflammation and are positively correlated with tumor progression and aggressiveness [53].

4. Exosomes for therapeutic intervention in cancer

The recent contribution by Zhang et al. reviewed the recent advances in cancer immunotherapy, exosome functions, exosome immunoregulation, and immune cell-derived exosomes [34]. As mentioned in Zhang's manuscript, exosomes cannot only transfer messages between cells by carrying RNA and proteins but also can modulate the immune response. After reviewing recent findings regarding exosomes and immunity in cancer, we have highlighted the novel insights into the development of efficient exosome-based cancer vaccines for cancer therapeutic intervention. Specifically, exosomes derived from immune cells, such as APCs, dendritic cells (DCs), and NK cells, play a crucial role in the immunomodulation of cancer, and they may be the best cancer vaccine candidates because they can inhibit the malignant activity of cancer cells and leave healthy cells unaffected [54–56]. Recently, researchers have noted that exosomes may lead to key advances in cancer therapy. Exosomes isolated from DCs have been evaluated in clinical trials as treatment for various kinds of cancers [57–59]. In a phase I clinical trial, exosomes derived from autologous DCs loaded with MAGE 3 peptides were applied as cancer therapy for stage III/IV melanoma patients [58]. Several phase I or phase II clinical trials involving exosome-based regimens have occurred in breast cancer, gastric cancer, malignant glioma, and non-small cell lung cancer patients, which demonstrates that exosomes are effective tools for the transportation of anticancer drugs [59]. Exosomes were employed to form a complex with curcumin and delivered to recipient pancreatic cancer cells, which was found to promote cytotoxicity [60]. Moreover, exosomes have been shown to deliver small, molecular anticancer drugs across the blood-brain barrier and significantly inhibit tumor growth in a brain cancer model [61, 62].

5. Long non-coding RNAs as novel biomarkers in cancer

lncRNAs modulate gene expression, while lncRNA dysregulation is associated with human cancer. lncRNAs could play a significant role in cancer progression by interacting with proteins. Since they are highly specific and easily detectable in tissue, serum, plasma, and urine, interest in exploring lncRNAs in cancer patients continues to increase. Metastasis-associated lung adenocarcinoma transcript 1 (MALAT-1, also known as NEAT2), a novel lncRNA, is found on chromosome 11q13 and is well conserved among mammalian species. MALAT-1 is a critical regulator of the metastatic phenotype of lung cancer cells [63] and can enhance proliferation, cell motility, invasion, and metastasis in CNE-1 [64], lung adenocarcinoma [65], thyroid cancer [17], cervical cancer [19], and ovarian cancer cells [18]. MALAT-1 has an important role in regulating the metastasis of bladder cancer and can be a potential application in bladder cancer therapy [66]. The MALAT-1-mediated promotion of renal cell carcinoma (RCC) proliferation and metastasis may be due to the upregulation of Livin expression [67]. MALAT-1 promotes the proliferation of chondrosarcoma cells via activating the Notch-1 signaling pathway [68], indicates poor prognosis in non-small cell lung cancer, and induces migration and tumor growth [69]. Upregulation of MALAT-1 has been associated with survival rate, cell cycle, and migration in patients with esophageal squamous cell carcinoma (ESCC) [70]. However, the loss of MALAT1 is compatible with cell viability and normal development [71]. On the other hand, MALAT-1 is downregulated in preeclampsia and regulates the proliferation, apoptosis, migration, and invasion of JEG-3 trophoblast cells [72]. MALAT-1 is also expected to be a potential therapeutic target in prostate cancer [73]. As another critical oncogenic lncRNA in human cancers [74, 75], the lncRNA HOTTIP promotes tumor growth, inhibits cell apoptosis [76], contributes to the progression of prostate cancer [77] and non-small cell lung cancer [78] by regulating HOXA13, and increases the chemoresistance of osteosarcoma cells by activating the Wnt/β-catenin pathway [79]. HOTTIP is upregulated and associated with poor prognosis in patients with osteosarcoma [80]. Overexpression of HOTTIP can promote tumor invasion and predict poor prognosis in gastric cancer [81]. This accumulating evidence indicates that long non-coding RNAs have immense potential as powerful, non-invasive tumor markers. However, overexpression of HOTTIP inhibits glioma cell growth by brain and reproductive expression [82].

Circulating lncRNAs have shown potential as biomarkers in the diagnosis and prognosis of many cancers, including cervical cancer, colon cancer, hepatocellular carcinoma (HCC), gastric cancer (GC), PaCa, renal cell carcinoma (RCC), ovarian cancer (OC), non-small cell lung cancer (NSCLC), thyroid cancer, and prostate cancer (**Table 1**). Here, we have identified some interesting circulating lncRNAs (also known as exosomal lncRNAs), including MALAT-1, PVT1, HOTAIR, H19, UCA1, and TUG1, as novel biomarkers in various cancers. MALAT-1 in urine may serve as a potential biomarker for predicting prostate cancer risk. The application of the MALAT-1 model can prevent 30.2–46.5% of unnecessary biopsies in high-grade cancers [83]. PVT1 expression has been shown to be significantly elevated in non-small cell lung cancer (NSCLC), and high PVT1 expression has been associated with poor overall survival and disease-free survival in NSCLC patients; therefore, PVT1 could serve as a promising biomarker for the diagnosis and prognosis of NSCLC. PVT1 knockdown could remarkably inhibit NSCLC cell proliferation [84]. HOTAIR has been shown to be significantly higher in breast cancer patients, and circulating HOTAIR DNA levels were 2.15-fold higher in patients compared with those of healthy controls in one study, which demonstrates a moderate correlation between its expressions in tumor tissues. Plasma HOTAIR levels have been found to be significantly reduced after surgery [85, 86], indicating that plasma HOTAIR might serve as a potential biomarker for diagnosing breast cancer. A multivariate survival analysis also

lncRNA	Functions	Detection in cancer	References
MALAT-1	1. Promotes cell proliferation, invasion, and migration	Thyroid cancer, OC, cervical cancer, NSCLC, human nasopharyngeal carcinoma cell lines, bladder cancer, lung adenocarcinoma, JEG-3 trophoblast cells, PaCa, chondrosarcoma cell, RCC, ESCC	[17–19, 66, 67, 71–75, 77, 106]
	2. Regulator of the metastasis	Lung cancer cells, human nasopharyngeal carcinoma cell lines, PaCa	[65, 66, 111]
	3. Diagnostic and prognostic biomarker	Prostate cancer (urine/ plasma), osteosarcoma (serum)	[78, 88, 123]
	4. Potential therapeutic target	Prostate cancer	[78]
HOTTIP	1. Inhibits glioma cell growth	Glioma	[87]
	2. Cell growth, apoptosis, migration, and invasion	HCC, PaCa, GC and colorectal cancer, NSCLC, lung cancer	[80, 81, 83, 85, 113, 123]
	3. Increases chemoresistance	Osteosarcoma cell, PaCa	[119]
	4. Progression and prognosis	Prostate cancer, colorectal cancer, osteosarcoma, tongue squamous cell carcinoma, PaCa, HCC	[80, 82, 119, 124–126]
	5. Biomarkers	PaCa (blood)	[121]
PVT1	1. Promotes cell proliferation and invasion	NSCLC, esophageal cancer, bladder cancer, acute promyelocytic leukemia, GC, BC	[127–133]
	2. Progression and prognosis	Cervical cancer, GC, HCC, PaCa	[115, 134–137]
	3. Promotes resistance	OC, GC	[138, 139]
	4. Modulates thyroid cancer cell proliferation	Thyroid cancer	[140]
	5. Apoptosis	Colorectal cancers	[141]
	6. Novel biomarker for diagnosis and prognosis	Cervical cancer, HCC, RCC (Serum); PaCa, NSCLC (tissue)	[89, 114, 142–145]
uc.345	1. Promotes tumorigenesis	PaCa	[122]
LINC-PINT	1. Diagnostic and prognostic biomarkers	PaCa (plasma and tumor tissues)	[127]

lncRNA	Functions	Detection in cancer	References
HOTAIR	1. Enhances cell proliferation, survival and migration	PaCa, HCC, cervical cancer, GC, OC, NSCLC, colorectal cancer, prostate cancer	[113, 146–155]
	2. Enhances its prognostic potential and correlates with disease progression	BC, HCC, cervical cancer, bladder cancer	[156–169]
	3. Relative to resistance	BC, cervical cancer, OC, bladder transitional cell carcinoma	[157, 160–162]
	4. Associated with EMT, cancer stem cells	Epithelial OC, colorectal cancer	[163, 164]
	5. Activates autophagy	HCC	[165]
	6. Modulates HLA-G expression	Cervical cancer, GC	[166, 167]
	7. Potential biomarker for diagnosis	PaCa, BC, colorectal carcinoma (serum/plasma), PaCa (tissue), GC (tissue, blood, and gastric juice)	[90, 91, 114, 149, 168–170]
H19	1. Promotes cell proliferation, migration and invasion	PDAC, lung cancer, BC, glioblastoma	[117, 172–174]
	2. Prognosis and progression and Metastasis	Gastrointestinal, colorectal cancer, NSCLC, gallbladder carcinoma	[175–179]
	3. Regulates angiogenesis	Glioma, glioblastoma	[173, 180]
	4. Contributing to resistance	OC	[181]
	5. Modulates tumorigenicity and stemness	Malignant carcinoma	[182]
	6. Regulatory role in pluripotency and tumorigenesis	Human embryonic carcinoma	[183]
	7. Promotes EMT	Colorectal cancer, esophageal cancer, glioblastoma	[173, 184, 185]
	8. Potential biomarkers for diagnosis	GC (serum/plasma/tissue), BC (tissue), bladder cancer	[91–93, 186–188]
IRAIN	1. Promotes proliferation and suppresses apoptosis	PaCa, NSCLC	[123, 189]
	2. As a novel imprinted gene that is aberrantly regulated in breast cancer	BC (tumors and peripheral blood leucocytes)	[190]

lncRNA	Functions	Detection in cancer	References
UCA1	1. Promotes the tumorigenesis, enhances cell proliferation, migration	PaCa, endometrial cancer, colorectal cancer, RCC, NSCLC, prostate cancer	[118, 191–194]
	2. Contributes to the progression and prognosis	OSCC, ESCC	[195, 196]
	3. Promotes EMT	BC	[197]
	4. Suppress metastasis	Epithelial OC	[198]
	5. Modulates cell growth and apoptosis, and epigenetic regulation	BC	[199, 200]
	6. Enhances drug resistance	BC, bladder cancer, GC, colorectal cancer, prostate cancer	[192, 201–205]
	7. Promotes glutamine metabolism	Bladder cancer	[206]
	8. As diagnostic and prognostic markers	HCC, colon cancer (serum), early gastric cancer, lung cancer (plasma), bladder cancer (urine and blood),	[171, 207–217]
TUG1	1. Promotes cell proliferation, migration	Bladder cancer, BC, osteosarcoma, ESCC, HCC	[218–222]
	2. Poor prognosis and promotes metastasis	Bladder cancer, GC, colorectal cancer, OC	[219, 223–226]
	3. Associated with chemotherapy resistance and poor prognosis	ESCC	[227]
	4. Acts as a tumor suppressor in human glioma	Human glioma	[228]
	5. Affects apoptosis and insulin secretion	PaCa	[124]
	6. As biomarker for poor prognosis	Osteosarcoma (plasma), B-cell neoplasms (plasma)	[229, 230]

Table 1. Long non-coding RNAs (lncRNAs) as potential biomarkers for cancer.

indicated that H19 might serve as a potential biomarker for early detection and prediction of prognosis of breast cancer and gastric cancer. The expression of H19 was remarkably increased in breast cancer and gastric cancer tissues. H19 expression has been shown to be significantly correlated with invasion depth, advanced TNM stage and regional lymph node metastasis in gastric cancer. Additionally, elevated expression levels of H19 have been shown to contribute to the poor overall survival and disease-free survival of gastric cancer patients [87]. This makes H19 closely associated with progressive gastric cancer, and it could be a potential non-invasive diagnostic gastric cancer biomarker for management. Better performance could be achieved using both carcinoembryonic antigen (CEA) and H19 simultaneously [88]. Plasma H19 levels have been shown to be significantly decreased in postoperative breast cancer samples compared to those in preoperative samples [89]. Urothelial cancer-associated 1 (UCA1), originally identified as a lncRNA in bladder cancer, has been proven to play a pivotal role in bladder cancer progression and embryonic development. Upregulation of the lncRNA UCA1 and the lncRNA WRAP53 has been observed in hepatocellular carcinoma (HCC), and CA1 might serve as a novel serum biomarker for HCC. Moreover, the expression levels of UCA1 and WRAP53 in tissue have been shown to be strongly correlated with their levels in sera. Further, the combination of UCA1 and WRAP53 with serum alpha fetoprotein could improve sensitivity to 100% [90]. Further, meta-analysis also found that higher levels of UCA1 were correlated with shorter progression-free survival (PFS) and overall survival (OS) times in cancer [91], indicating that circulating lncRNAs, such as MALAT-1, PVT1, HOTAIR, H19, UCA1, and WRAP53, could serve as novel biomarkers for the early detection and the prediction of prognosis of cancer.

6. Exosomes and lncRNAs in the diagnosis and treatment of pancreatic cancer

Pancreatic cancer is one of the most lethal tumors, and its main tumor type is that of adenocarcinoma [92–94]. Pancreatic ductal adenocarcinoma (PDAC), the fourth leading cause of cancer-related deaths in both males and females in the USA, is usually asymptomatic [186], and PDAC is one of the most lethal malignant neoplasms worldwide [89, 95, 96]. Statistical analysis indicated that death rates rose from 2001 to 2010 [97]. In America, approximately 53,000 people were diagnosed with pancreatic cancer in 2016, and pancreatic cancer was responsible for 41,750 deaths in the USA [98] in that same year. Additionally, the incidence of pancreatic cancer has shown an increasing trend year-by-year in China, and pancreatic cancer has become one of the top 10 causes of cancer-related deaths [99].

It is well known that pancreatic cancer has a poor prognosis because it is usually diagnosed after the cancer has already spread, leading to poor patient outcomes. Pancreatic ductal adenocarcinoma patients have a 5-year survival rate of ~5% [100]. Survival can be improved if tumors are detected at an early stage, and the 5-year survival rate is 50% if tumors are <2 cm in size [101]. However, there have been no reliable biomarkers to accurately diagnose, image, or predict the tumor classification and biological behavior of pancreatic cancer until now. Thus, it is urgent to screen potential biomarkers and treatment-related biomarkers, such as exosome-derived proteins, DNA (exoDNA), miRNAs (exosomal miRNAs), and lncRNAs (exosomal lncRNAs), for the early detection of pancreatic cancer. Allenson found that KRAS mutations in the exoDNA of control, localized, locally advanced, and metastatic PDAC patients were 7.4, 66.7, 80, and 85%, respectively, which demonstrates that KRAS in exosomes could be applied to diagnose PDAC [102]. Takikawa also confirmed that pancreatic stellate cell (PSC)-derived exosomes stimulate the proliferation and migration of pancreatic cancer cells and upregulate the mRNA expression of the chemokine (C-X-C motif) ligands 1 and 2 in pancreatic cancer cells [103]. Over the last few years, non-coding RNAs, especially exosomal lncRNAs and exosomal miRNAs, have become a new diagnostic, prognostic, and predictive tool for pancreatic cancer. Exosomal miR-155, miR-196a, miR-17-5p, miR-10b, and miR-21 have good sensitivity and specificity in the serum of PaCa patients and can be useful serum biomarkers for pancreatic cancer [104, 105]. Not only can single exosomes be a diagnosis biomarker, but combined exosomal miRNAs, such as miR-1246, miR-4644, miR-3976, and miR-4306, can also increase sensitivity and specificity for the diagnosis of pancreatic cancer.

Specifically, exosomal lncRNAs have been identified as potential biomarkers of various cancers in recent years, including gastric cancer, breast cancer, and lung cancer. However, few studies have explored the potential use of exosomal lncRNAs in pancreatic cancer detection and prognosis. MALAT-1, HOTTIP, PVT1, and HOTAIR, which are secreted from PDAC cells to bodily fluids, such as blood, pancreatic juice, cystic fluid, and urine, are some of most widely studied lncRNAs in pancreatic cancer (**Figure 1**). As a potential oncogenic lncRNA, MALAT-1 involves in proliferation, migration, and invasion and promotes the undifferentiated phenotype of pancreatic tumor cells [106]. MALAT-1 can also promote the tumorigenicity of pancreatic cancer cells, increase the proportion of pancreatic cancer stem cells, maintain a self-renewing capacity, and decrease chemosensitivity to anticancer drugs. Moreover, MALAT-1 has potential effects on the stem cell-like phenotypes of pancreatic cancer cells, which suggests that MALAT-1 has a novel role in tumor stemness [107]. The lncRNA HOTTIP enhances pancreatic cancer cell proliferation, survival, and migration and has been implicated in pancreatic cancer diagnosis and prognosis [108]. The overexpression of HOTAIR has been described as a poor prognostic factor in PDAC and can also be a novel non-invasive salivary biomarker for the early diagnosis of PaCa with PVT1 expression [109]. Increased expression of the lncRNA PVT1 is associated with poor prognosis in pancreatic cancer patients [110]. PVT1 expression is

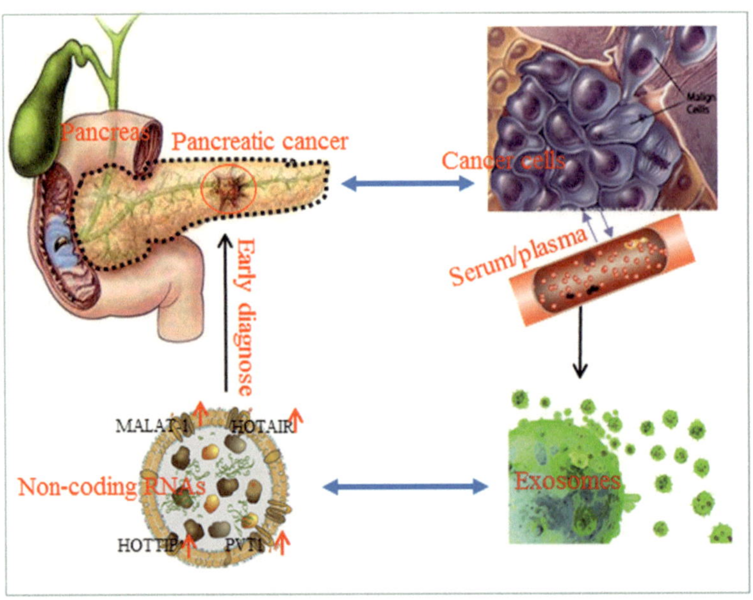

Figure 1. Exosomal lncRNAs secreted from PDAC cells as potential biomarkers of pancreatic cancer.

significantly increased in PDAC and is correlated with tumor progression. Moreover, patients with high PVT1 expression levels have been shown to have shorter overall survival times compared to those with low PVT1 expression levels, which implies that PVT1 could be a potential molecular biomarker for predicting the prognosis of patients with PDAC [110]. H19 has been shown to be overexpressed in PDAC tissues and to be correlated with the histological grade of PDAC. Knockdown of H19 can suppress cell viability, proliferation, and tumor growth, while H19 overexpression can enhance cell viability, proliferation, and tumor growth [111]. UCA1 expression has been shown to be significantly upregulated in PaCa tumor tissues and to be significantly correlated with malignant potential factors, such as tumor size, depth of invasion, CA19-9 levels, and tumor stage. Highly expressed UCA1 has been shown to be an independent prognostic biomarker of PaCa, leading to an obviously shorter 5-year overall survival (OS). Downregulation of UCA1 could effectively inhibit cell proliferative activities, which implies that UCA1 could be a potential prognostic biomarker and therapy target of PaCa [112].

In addition, high expression levels of the lncRNA HOXA13 have been shown to be correlated with lymph node metastasis, poor histological differentiation, and decreased overall survival in PDAC patients. The knockdown of HOXA13 resulted in proliferation arrest and impaired cell invasion in pancreatic cancer [113]. Using microarray analysis, HOTTIP was confirmed to be one of the most significantly upregulated lncRNAs in PDAC [113]. HOTTIP has been shown to be overexpressed in pancreatic cancer, and knockdown of HOTTIP in pancreatic cancer cells decreased proliferation, induced apoptosis, and decreased migration [108]. Using an Arraystar Human lncRNA Microarray, HOTTIP-005, XLOC_006390, and RP11-567G11.1 were found to be the most increased lncRNAs in PaCa. Elevated HOTTIP-005 and RP11-567G11.1 expression could serve as poor prognostic markers for patients with PaCa. Plasma HDRF and RDRF (HOTTIP-005- and RP11-567G11.1-derived RNA fragments in plasma/serum) have also shown to be significantly increased in patients with PaCa, which demonstrates that HDRF and RDRF levels could be promising indicators for distinguishing patients with PC [114]. As an oncogenic lncRNA, uc.345 has been shown to promote tumor progression and to serve as a poor predictor for OS in pancreatic cancer patients. uc.345 was found to be upregulated in tumor tissues, and higher uc.345 expression levels have been associated with cancer invasion and metastasis, which could be an independent risk factor for the OS of pancreatic cancer patients [115]. The lncRNA IRAIN plays an important role in many malignancies, and upregulation of IRAIN has been shown to be significantly correlated with tumor size, the TNM classification of malignant tumors (TNM) stage, and lymph node metastasis in PaCa patients. The knockdown of IRAIN significantly induced cell apoptosis and inhibited cell proliferation in PaCa cells [116]. The lncRNA TUG1 has been shown to be highly expressed in pancreatic tissue compared with its expression in other organ tissues, and downregulation of TUG1 has been shown to affect apoptosis and insulin secretion in pancreatic β cells [117]. CCDC26 might be identified as a novel oncogene in PaCa by regulating proliferating cell nuclear antigen (PCNA) and Bcl2 expression. CCDC26 is significantly upregulated in PaCa, and it is correlated with tumor size, tumor number, and reduced OS [118]. Univariate and multivariate analysis showed that CCDC26 expression can be an independent prognostic factor of OS in patients with PaCa; therefore, CCDC2 could serve as a novel biomarker and therapeutic target of PC for cancer in the future [118]. LINC-ROR has been shown to be upregulated in PaCa tissues, and overexpression of LINC-ROR promoted cell proliferation, migration, invasion, and metastasis both in vitro and in mouse models. LINC-ROR acts as an important regulator of ZEB1 and might represent a novel therapeutic target [119]. The lncRNA LINC-PINT (p53-induced transcript) could also regulate tumor cell viability and proliferation. However, the expression levels of LINC-PINT have been shown to be lower in plasma and tumor tissue samples in PaCa patients. LINC-PINT has been shown to be more sensitive than CA19-9 in detecting PaCa, which suggests that LINC-PINT could be used for distinguishing the cause of malignant obstructive jaundice [120]. The lncRNA HMlincRNA717 has also been shown to be downregulated in pancreatic cancer and associated with overall survival, suggesting that HMlincRNA717 could be a potential prognostic biomarker for pancreatic cancer progression [121]. As a potential tumor suppressor, the long intergenic non-coding RNA (lincRNA) LINC00673 has been associated with pancreatic cancer risk. A G>A mutation at rs11655237 of LINC00673 created a target site for miR-1231 binding, which diminished the effect of LINC00673 in an allele-specific manner and conferred susceptibility to PaCa [122].

All the abovementioned exosomal lncRNAs could serve as diagnostic and prognostic factors to complement clinical and pathological parameters in predicting the outcome of patients with pancreatic cancer. Although there are an increasing number of clinical assays for studying exosomes, determining clinical applications for lncRNAs and exosomes is a long ways off. No matter how exosomes have become the most effective cancer vaccines, future research to investigate exosomal lncRNAs as biomarkers for the early detection of pancreatic cancer and to assess the validity and quality of the exosomes as effective vaccines for pancreatic cancer will be valuable. To achieve this long-term goal, further understanding of exosome biology, especially of the molecular mechanisms of tumor- and immune cell-derived exosomes as cancer vaccines, is required.

Acknowledgement

This research was supported by a grant from the National Natural Science Foundation of China (81672383) and a grant (16PJ1408800) from the Shanghai Pujiang Program in Shanghai, China.

Abbreviations

APC	Antigen-presenting cell
BC	Breast cancer
BPH	Benign prostatic hyperplasia
CEA	Carcinoembryonic antigen
DCs	Dendritic cells
EMT	Epithelial-mesenchymal transition
EOC	Epithelial ovarian cancer
ESCC	Esophageal squamous cell carcinoma
EVs	Extracellular vesicles
GC	Gastric cancer

HCC	Hepatocellular carcinoma
PCNA	Proliferating cell nuclear antigen
PFS	Progression-free survival
lncRNAs	Long non-coding RNAs
MALAT-1	Metastasis-associated lung adenocarcinoma transcript 1
ncRNAs	Non-coding RNAs
NSCLC	Non-small cell lung cancer
OC	Ovarian cancer
OS	Overall survival
OSCC	Oral squamous cell carcinoma
PaCa	Pancreatic cancer
PDAC	Pancreatic ductal adenocarcinoma
RCC	Renal cell carcinoma
sncRNAs	Small ncRNAs
UCA1	Urothelial cancer-associated 1

Author details

Jin Wang[1]*, Xuan Zhang[1], Chunxia Ji[1], Lei Zhang[2], Yang Di[3], Wenhui Lou[2], Xiaoyan Zhang[1] and Jianqing Xu[1]

*Address all correspondence to: wangjin@shaphc.org

1 Scientific Research Center, Shanghai Public Health Clinical Center, Fudan University, Shanghai, China

2 General Surgery Department, Zhongshan Hospital, Fudan University, Shanghai, China

3 Department of Pancreatic Surgery, Pancreatic Disease Institute, Huashan Hospital, Shanghai Medical College, Fudan University, Shanghai, China

References

[1] Tkach M, Thery C. Communication by extracellular vesicles: Where we are and where we need to go. Cell. 2016;**164**:1226-1232

[2] Thery C, Zitvogel L, Amigorena S. Exosomes: Composition, biogenesis and function. Nature Reviews Immunology. 2002;**2**:569-579

[3] Keller S, Sanderson MP, Stoeck A, Altevogt P. Exosomes: From biogenesis and secretion to biological function. Immunology Letters. 2006;**107**(2):102-108

[4] Nuzhat Z, Kinhal V, Sharma S, Rice GE, Joshi V, Salomon C. Tumour-derived exosomes as a signature of pancreatic cancer—liquid biopsies as indicators of tumour progression. Oncotarget. 2017;**8**(10):17279-17291

[5] Clombo M, Raposo G, Thery C. Biogenesis, secretion, and intercellular interactions of exosomes and other extracellular vesicles. Annual Review of Cell and Developmental Biology. 2014;**30**:255-289

[6] Raposo G, Stoorvogel W. Extracellular vesicles: Exosomes, microvesicles, and friends. The Journal of Cell Biology. 2013;**200**(4):373-383

[7] Brinton LT, Sloane HS, Kester M, Kelly KA. Formation and role of exosomes in cancer. Cellular and Molecular Life Sciences. 2015;**72**(4):659-671

[8] Costa-Silva B, Aiello NM, Ocean AJ, Singh S, Zhang H, Thakur BK, et al. Pancreatic cancer exosomes initiate pre-metastatic niche formation in the liver. Nature Cell Biology. 2015;**17**(6):816-826

[9] Hoshino A, Costa-Silva B, Shen TL, Rodrigues G, Hashimoto A, Tesic Mark M, et al. Tumour exosome integrins determine organotropic metastasis. Nature. 2015;**527**(7578):329-335

[10] Peinado H, Aleckovic M, Lavotshkin S, Matei I, Costa-Silva B, Moreno-Bueno G, et al. Melanoma exosomes educate bone marrow progenitor cells toward a pro-metastatic phenotype through MET. Nature Medicine. 2012;**18**(6):883-891

[11] Valadi H, Ekstrom K, Bossios A, Sjöstrand M, Lee JJ, Lötvall JO. Exosome-mediated transfer of mRNAs and microRNAs is a novel mechanism of genetic exchange between cells. Nature Cell Biology. 2007;**9**(6):654-659

[12] Esteller M. Non-coding RNAs in human disease. Nature Reviews Genetics. 2011;**12**(12):861-874

[13] Lee JT. Epigenetic regulation by long noncoding RNAs. Science. 2012;**338**(6113):1435-1439

[14] Wapinski O, Chang HY. Long noncoding RNAs and human disease. Trends in Cell Biology. 2011;**21**(6):354-361

[15] Hung T, Chang HY. Long noncoding RNA in genome regulation: Prospects and mechanisms. RNA Biology. 2010;**7**(5):582-585

[16] Guttman M, Amit I, Garber M, French C, Lin MF, Feldser D, et al. Chromatin signature reveals over a thousand highly conserved large non-coding RNAs in mammals. Nature. 2009;**458**(7235):223-227

[17] Huang JK, Ma L, Song WH, Lu BY, Huang YB, Dong HM, et al. MALAT1 promotes the proliferation and invasion of thyroid cancer cells via regulating the expression of IQGAP1. Biomedicine & Pharmacotherapy. 2016;**83**:1-7

[18] Zhou Y, Xu X, Lv H, Wen Q, Li J, Tan L, et al. The long noncoding RNA MALAT-1 is highly expressed in ovarian cancer and induces cell growth and migration. PLoS One. 2016;**11**(5):e0155250

[19] Zhang Y, Wang T, Huang HQ, Li W, Cheng XL, Yang J. Human MALAT-1 long non-coding RNA is overexpressed in cervical cancer metastasis and promotes cell proliferation, invasion and migration. Journal of BUON. 2015;**20**(6):1497-1503

[20] Kino T, Hurt DE, Ichijo T, Nader N, Chrousos GP. Noncoding RNA gas5 is a growth arrest- and starvation-associated repressor of the glucocorticoid receptor. Science Signaling. 2010;**3**(107):ra8

[21] Hu W, Yuan B, Flygare J, Lodish HF. Long noncoding RNA-mediated anti-apoptotic activity in murine erythroid terminal differentiation. Genes and Development. 2011;**25**(24):2573-2578

[22] Meola N, Pizzo M, Alfano G, Surace EM, Banfi S. The long noncoding RNA Vax2os1 controls the cell cycle progression of photoreceptor progenitors in the mouse retina. RNA. 2012;**18**(1):111-123

[23] Tripathi V, Ellis JD, Shen Z, Song DY, Pan Q, Watt AT, et al. The nuclear-retained noncoding RNA MALAT1 regulates alternative splicing by modulating SR splicing factor phosphorylation. Molecular Cell. 2010;**39**(6):925-938

[24] Wang KC, Yang YW, Liu B, Sanyal A, Corces-Zimmerman R, Chen Y, et al. A long noncoding RNA maintains active chromatin to coordinate homeotic gene expression. Nature. 2011;**472**(7341):120-124

[25] Tsai MC, Manor O, Wan Y, Mosammaparast N, Wang JK, Lan F, et al. Long noncoding RNA as modular scaffold of histone modification complexes. Science. 2010;**329**(5992):689-693

[26] Loewer S, Cabili MN, Guttman M, Loh YH, Thomas K, Park IH, et al. Large intergenic non-coding RNA-RoR modulates reprogramming of human induced pluripotent stem cells. Nature Genetics. 2010;**42**(12):1113-1117

[27] Guttman M, Donaghey J, Carey BW, Garber M, Grenier JK, Munson G, et al. lincRNAs act in the circuitry controlling pluripotency and differentiation. Nature. 2011;**477**(7364):295-300

[28] Gregg C, Zhang J, Weissbourd B, Luo S, Schroth GP, Haig D, et al. High-resolution analysis of parent-of-origin allelic expression in the mouse brain. Science. 2010;**329**(5992):643-648

[29] EL Andaloussi S, Mäger I, Breakefield XO, Wood MJ. Extracellular vesicles: Biology and emerging therapeutic opportunities. Nature Reviews Drug Discovery. 2013;**12**(5):347-357

[30] De Toro J, Herschlik L, Waldner C, Mongini C. Emerging roles of exosomes in normal and pathological conditions: New insights for diagnosis and therapeutic applications. Frontiers in Immunology. 2015;**4**(6):203

[31] Meckes DG. Exosomal communication goes viral. Journal of Virology. 2015;**89**(10):5200-5203

[32] Barteneva NS, Maltsev N, Vorobjev IA. Microvesicles and intercellular communication in the context of parasitism. Frontiers in Cellular and Infection Microbiology. 2013;**6**(3):49

[33] Kucharzewska P, Belting M. Emerging roles of extracellular vesicles in the adaptive response of tumour cells to microenvironmental stress. Journal of Extracellular Vesicles. 2013. DOI: 10.3402/jev.v2i0.20304

[34] Zhang X, Pei Z, Chen J, Ji C, Xu J, Zhang X, et al. Exosomes for immunoregulation and therapeutic intervention in cancer. Journal of Cancer. 2016;**7**(9):1081-1087

[35] Runz S, Keller S, Rupp C, Stoeck A, Issa Y, Koensgen D, et al. Malignant ascites-derived exosomes of ovarian carcinoma patients contain CD24 and EpCAM. Gynecologic Oncology. 2007;**107**(3):563-571

[36] Simons M, Raposo G. Exosomes—Vesicular carriers for intercellular communication. Current Opinion in Cell Biology. 2009;**21**(4):578-581

[37] Kowal J, Tkach M, Théry C. Biogenesis and secretion of exosomes. Current Opinion in Cell Biology. 2014;**29**:116-125

[38] Mathivana S, Ji H, Simpson RJ. Exosomes: Extracellular organelles important in intercellular communication. Journal of Proteomics. 2010;**73**(10):1907-1920

[39] Wolfers J, Lozier A, Raposo G, Regnault A, Théry C, Masurier C, et al. Tumor-derived exosomes are a source of shared tumor rejection antigens for CTL cross-priming. Nature Medicine. 2001;**7**(3):297-303

[40] Chiba M, Kimura M, Asari S. Exosomes secreted from human colorectal cancer cell lines contain mRNAs, microRNAs and natural antisense RNAs, that can transfer into the human hepatoma HepG2 and lung cancer A549 cell lines. Oncology Reports. 2012;**28**(5):1551-1558

[41] Wu L, Zhang X, Zhang B, Shi H, Yuan X, Sun Y, et al. Exosomes derived from gastric cancer cells activate NF-κB pathway in macrophages to promote cancer progression. Tumour Biology. 2016;**37**(9):12169-12180

[42] Nakamura K, Sawada K, Kinose Y, Yoshimura A, Toda A, Nakatsuka E, et al. Exosomes promote ovarian cancer cell invasion through transfer of CD44 to peritoneal mesothelial cells. Mol Cancer Res. 2017;**5**(1):78-92

[43] Melo SA, Luecke LB, Kahlert C, Fernandez AF, Gammon ST, Kaye J, et al. Glypican-1 identifies cancer exosomes and detects early pancreatic cancer. Nature. 2015;**523**(7559):177-182

[44] Rupp AK, Rupp C, Keller S, Brase JC, Ehehalt R, Fogel M, et al. Loss of EpCAM expression in breast cancer derived serum exosomes: Role of proteolytic cleavage. Gynecologic Oncology. 2011;**122**(2):437-446

[45] Moon PG, Lee JE, Cho YE, Lee SJ, Chae YS, Jung JH, et al. Fibronectin on circulating extracellular vesicles as a liquid biopsy to detect breast cancer. Oncotarget. 2016;**7**(26): 40189-40199

[46] Moon PG, Lee JE, Cho YE, Lee SJ, Jung JH, Chae YS, et al. Identification of developmental endothelial locus-1 on circulating extracellular vesicles as a novel biomarker for early breast cancer detection. Clinical Cancer Research. 2016;**22**(7):1757-1766

[47] Khan S, Jutzy JMS, Valenzuela MMA, Turay D, Aspe JR, Ashok A, et al. Plasma-derived exosomal survivin, a plausible biomarker for early detection of prostate cancer. PLoS One. 2012;**7**(10):e46737

[48] Ratajczak J, Wysoczynski M, Hayek F, Janowska-Wieczorek A, Ratajczak MZ. Membranederived microvesicles: Important and underappreciated mediators of cell-to-cell communication. Leukemia. 2006;**20**(9):1487-1495

[49] Gusachenko ON, Zenkova MA, Vlassov VV. Nucleic acids in exosomes: Disease markers and intercellular communication molecules. Biochemistry (Moscow). 2013;**78**(1):1-7

[50] Bullock MD, Silva AM, Kanlikilicer P, Filant J, Rashed MH, Sood AK, et al. Exosomal non-coding RNAs: Diagnostic, prognostic and therapeutic applications in cancer. Non-Coding RNA. 2015;**1**:53-68

[51] Zhou X, Wen W, Shan X, Zhu W, Xu J, Guo R, et al. A six-microRNA panel in plasma was identified as a potential biomarker for lung adenocarcinoma diagnosis. Oncotarget. 2017;**8**(4):6513-6525

[52] Taylor DD, Gercel-Taylor C. MicroRNA signatures of tumor-derived exosomes as diagnostic biomarkers of ovarian cancer. Gynecologic Oncology. 2008;**110**(1):13-21

[53] Tanaka Y, Kamohara H, Kinoshita K, Kurashige J, Ishimoto T, Iwatsuki M, et al. Clinical impact of serum exosomal microRNA-21 as a clinical biomarker in human esophageal squamous cell carcinoma. Cancer. 2013;**119**(6):1159-1167

[54] Zitvogel L, Regnault A, Lozier A, Wolfers J, Flament C, Tenza D, et al. Eradication of established murine tumors using a novel cell-free vaccine: Dendritic cell derived exosomes. Nature Medicine. 1998;**4**(5):594-600

[55] Baleeiro RB, Anselmo LB, Soares FA, Pinto CA, Ramos O, Gross JL, et al. High frequency of immature dendritic cells and altered in situ production of interleukin-4 and tumor necrosis factor-alpha in lung cancer. Cancer Immunology, Immunotherapy. 2008;**57**(9):1335-1345

[56] Thery C, Regnault A, Garin J, Wolfers J, Zitvogel L, Ricciardi-Castagnoli P, et al. Molecular characterization of dendritic cell derived exosomes. Selective accumulation of the heat shock protein hsc73. The Journal of Cell Biology. 1999;**147**(3):599-610

[57] Viaud S, Thery C, Ploix S. Dendritic cell-derived exosomes for cancer immunotherapy: What's next? Cancer Research. 2010;**70**(4):1281-1285

[58] Escudier B, Dorval T, Chaput N, André F, Caby MP, Novault S, et al. Vaccination of metastatic melanoma patients with autologous dendritic cell (DC) derived-exosomes: Results of the first phase I clinical trial. Journal of Translational Medicine. 2005;**3**(1):10

[59] Azmi AS, Bao B, Sarkar FH. Exosomes in cancer development, metastasis, and drug resistance: A comprehensive review. Cancer Metastasis Reviews. 2013;**32**(3-4):623-642

[60] Osterman CJ, Lynch JC, Leaf P, Gonda A, Ferguson Bennit HR, Griffiths D, et al. Curcumin modulates pancreatic adenocarcinoma cell-derived exosomal function. PLoS One. 2015;| **10**(7):e0132845

[61] Pardridge WM. Drug transport across the blood–brain barrier. Journal of Cerebral Blood Flow and Metabolism. 2012;**32**(11):1959-1972

[62] Yang T, Martin P, Fogarty B, Brown A, Schurman K, Phipps R, et al. Exosome delivered anticancer drugs across the blood-brain barrier for brain cancer therapy in *Danio rerio*. Pharmaceutical Research. 2015;**32**(6):2003-2014

[63] Gutschner T, Hammerle M, Diederichs S. MALAT1—a paradigm for long noncoding RNA function in cancer. Journal of Molecular Medicine. 2013;**91**(7):791-801

[64] Xie L, Hu Z, Wang X, Li Z. Expression of long noncoding RNA MALAT1 gene in human nasopharyngeal carcinoma cell lines and its biological significance. Nan Fang Yi Ke Da Xue Xue Bao. 2013;**33**(5):692-697

[65] Tano K, Mizuno R, Okada T, Rakwal R, Shibato J, Masuo Y, et al. MALAT-1 enhances cell motility of lung adenocarcinoma cells by influencing the expression of motility-related genes. FEBS Letters. 2010;**584**(22):4575-4580

[66] Ying L, Chen Q, Wang Y, Zhou Z, Huang Y, Qiu F. Upregulated MALAT-1 contributes to bladder cancer cell migration by inducing epithelial-to-mesenchymal transition. Molecular Biosystems. 2012;**8**(9):2289-2294

[67] Chen S, Ma P, Zhao Y, Li B, Jiang S, Xiong H, et al. Biological function and mechanism of MALAT-1 in renal cell carcinoma proliferation and apoptosis: Role of the MALAT-1-Livin protein interaction. The Journal of Physiological Sciences. 2016. DOI: 10.1007/s12576-016-0486-8.

[68] Xu F, Zhang ZQ, Fang YC, Li XL, Sun Y, Xiong CZ, et al. Metastasis-associated lung adenocarcinoma transcript 1 promotes the proliferation of chondrosarcoma cell via activating Notch-1 signaling pathway. OncoTargets and Therapy. 2016;**9**:2143-2151

[69] Schmidt LH, Spieker T, Koschmieder S, Schäffers S, Humberg J, Jungen D, et al. The long noncoding MALAT-1 RNA indicates a poor prognosis in non-small cell lung cancer and induces migration and tumor growth. Journal of Thoracic Oncology. 2011;**6**(12):1984-1992

[70] Yao W, Bai Y, Li Y, Guo L, Zeng P, Wang Y, et al. Upregulation of MALAT-1 and its association with survival rate and the effect on cell cycle and migration in patients with esophageal squamous cell carcinoma. Tumour Biology. 2016;**37**(4):4305-4312

[71] Eißmann M, Gutschner T, Hämmerle M, Günther S, Caudron-Herger M, Groß M, et al. Loss of the abundant nuclear non-coding RNA MALAT1 is compatible with life and development.RNA Biology. 2012;**9**(8):1076-1087

[72] Chen H, Meng T, Liu X, Sun M, Tong C, Liu J, et al. Long non-coding RNA MALAT-1 is downregulated in preeclampsia and regulates proliferation, apoptosis, migration and invasion of JEG-3 trophoblast cells. International Journal of Clinical and Experimental Pathology. 2015;**8**(10):12718-12727

[73] Ren S, Liu Y, Xu W, Sun Y, Lu J, Wang F, et al. Long noncoding RNA MALAT-1 is a new potential therapeutic target for castration resistant prostate cancer. The Journal of Urology. 2013;**190**(6):2278-2287

[74] Lian Y, Cai Z, Gong H, Xue S, Wu D, Wang K. HOTTIP: A critical oncogenic long non-coding RNA in human cancers. Molecular Biosystems. 2016;**12**(11):3247-3253

[75] Chang S, Liu J, Guo S, He S, Qiu G, Lu J, et al. HOTTIP and HOXA13 are oncogenes associated with gastric cancer progression. Oncology Reports. 2016;**35**(6):3577-3585

[76] Deng HP, Chen L, Fan T, Zhang B, Xu Y, Geng Q. Long non-coding RNA HOTTIP promotes tumor growth and inhibits cell apoptosis in lung cancer. Cellular and Molecular Biology (Noisy-le-Grand, France). 2015;**61**(4):34-40

[77] Zhang SR, Yang JK, Xie JK, Zhao LC. Long noncoding RNA HOTTIP contributes to the progression of prostate cancer by regulating HOXA13. Cellular and Molecular Biology (Noisy-le-Grand, France). 2016;**62**(3):84-88

[78] Sang Y, Zhou F, Wang D, Bi X, Liu X, Hao Z, et al. Up-regulation of long non-coding HOTTIP functions as an oncogene by regulating HOXA13 in non-small cell lung cancer. American Journal of Translational Research. 2016;**8**(5):2022-2032

[79] Li Z, Zhao L, Wang Q. Overexpression of long non-coding RNA HOTTIP increases chemoresistance of osteosarcoma cell by activating the Wnt/β-catenin pathway. American Journal of Translational Research. 2016;**8**(5):2385-2393

[80] Li F, Cao L, Hang D, Wang F, Wang Q. Long non-coding RNA HOTTIP is up-regulated and associated with poor prognosis in patients with osteosarcoma. International Journal of Clinical and Experimental Pathology. 2015;**8**(9):11414-11420

[81] Ye H, Liu K, Qian K. Overexpression of long noncoding RNA HOTTIP promotes tumor invasion and predicts poor prognosis in gastric cancer. OncoTargets and Therapy. 2016;**9**:2081-2088

[82] Xu LM, Chen L, Li F, Zhang R, Li ZY, Chen FF, et al. Over-expression of the long non-coding RNA HOTTIP inhibits glioma cell growth by BRE. Journal of Experimental & Clinical Cancer Research. 2016;**35**(1):162

[83] Wang F, Ren S, Chen R, Lu J, Shi X, Zhu Y, et al. Development and prospective multicenter evaluation of the long noncoding RNA MALAT-1 as a diagnostic urinary biomarker for prostate cancer. Oncotarget. 2014;**5**(22):11091-11102

[84] Cui D, Yu CH, Liu M, Xia QQ, Zhang YF, Jiang WL. Long non-coding RNA PVT1 as a novel biomarker for diagnosis and prognosis of non-small cell lung cancer. Tumour Biology. 2016;**37**(3):4127-4134

[85] Zhang KJ, Zhang Y, Luo ZL, Liu L, Yang J, Wu LC, et al. Long non-coding RNA HOTAIR in plasma as a potential biomarker for breast cancer diagnosis. Nan Fang Yi Ke Da Xue Xue Bao. 2016;**36**(4):488-492

[86] Zhang L, Song X, Wang X, Xie Y, Wang Z, Xu Y, et al. Circulating DNA of HOTAIR in serum is a novel biomarker for breast cancer. Breast Cancer Research and Treatment. 2015;**152**(1):199-208

[87] Chen JS, Wang YF, Zhang XQ, Lv JM, Li Y, Liu XX, et al. H19 serves as a diagnostic biomarker and up-regulation of H19 expression contributes to poor prognosis in patients with gastric cancer. Neoplasma. 2016;**63**(2):223-230

[88] Hashad D, Elbanna A, Ibrahim A, Khedr G. Evaluation of the role of circulating long non-coding RNA H19 as a promising novel biomarker in plasma of patients with gastric cancer. Journal of Clinical Laboratory Analysis. 2016;**30**(6):1100-1105

[89] Zhang K, Luo Z, Zhang Y, Zhang L, Wu L, Liu L, et al. Circulating lncRNA H19 in plasma as a novel biomarker for breast cancer. Cancer Biomarkers. 2016;**17**(2):187-194

[90] Kamel MM, Matboli M, Sallam M, Montasser IF, Saad AS, El-Tawdi AH. Investigation of long noncoding RNAs expression profile as potential serum biomarkers in patients with hepatocellular carcinoma. Translational Research. 2016;**168**:134-145

[91] Hong HH, Hou LK, Pan X, Wu CY, Huang H, Li B, et al. Long non-coding RNA UCA1 is a predictive biomarker of cancer. Oncotarget. 2016;**7**(28):44442-44447

[92] Ferlay J, Soerjomataram I, Ervik M, Dikshit R, Eser S, Mathers C, et al. Cancer Incidence and Mortality Worldwide: IARC CancerBase No. 11. Lyon, France: International Agency for Research on Cancer; 2013

[93] Hidalgo M, Cascinu S, Kleeff J, Labianca R, Löhr JM, Neoptolemos J, et al. Addressing the challenges of pancreatic cancer: Future directions for improving outcomes. Pancreatology. 2013;**15**(1):8-18

[94] Vincent A, Herman J, Schulick R, Hruban RH, Goggins M. Pancreatic cancer. Lancet. 2011;**378**(9791):607-620

[95] Ferlay J, Soerjomataram I, Dikshit R, Eser S, Mathers C, Rebelo M, et al. Cancer incidence and mortality worldwide: Sources, methods and major patterns in GLOBOCAN. International Journal of Cancer. 2015;**136**(5):E359–E386

[96] Howlader N, Noone AM, Krapcho M, Miller D, Bishop K, Altekruse SF, et al. SEER Cancer Statistics Review, 1975-2013. Bethesda, MD: National Cancer Institute; 2016

[97] Siegel R, Ma J, Zou Z, Jemal A. Cancer statistics, 2014. CA: A Cancer Journal for Clinicians. 2014;**64**(1):9-29

[98] Hanada K, Okazaki A, Hirano N, Izumi Y, Teraoka Y, Ikemoto J, et al. Diagnostic strategies for early pancreatic cancer. Journal of Gastroenterology. 2015;**50**(2):147-154

[99] Chen W, Zheng R, Baade PD, et al. Cancer statistics in China, 2015. CA: A Cancer Journal for Clinicians. 2016;**66**(2):115-132

[100] Siegel RL, Miller KD, Jemal A. Cancer Statistics, 2017. CA Cancer J Clin. 2017 Jan;**67** (1):7-30

[101] Egawa S, Takeda K, Fukuyama S, Motoi F, Sunamura M, Matsuno S. Clinicopathological aspects of small pancreatic cancer. Pancreas. 2004;**28**(3):235-240

[102] Allenson K, Castillo J, San Lucas FA, Scelo G, Kim DU, Bernard V, et al. High prevalence of mutant KRAS in circulating exosome-derived DNA from early stage pancreatic cancer patients. Annals of Oncology. 2017;**28**(4):741-747

[103] Takikawa T, Masamune A, Yoshida N, Hamada S, Kogure T, Shimosegawa T. Exosomes derived from pancreatic stellate cells: MicroRNA signature and effects on pancreatic cancer cells. Pancreas. 2017;**46**(1):19-27

[104] Que R, Ding G, Chen J, Cao L. Analysis of serum exosomal microRNAs and clinicopathologic features of patients with pancreatic adenocarcinoma. World Journal of Surgical Oncology. 2013;**11**:219

[105] Joshi GK, Deitz-McElyea S, Liyanage T, Lawrence K, Mali S, Sardar R, et al. Labelfree nanoplasmonic-based short noncoding RNA sensing at attomolar concentrations allows for quantitative and highly specific assay of microRNA-10b in biological fluids and circulating exosomes. ACS Nano. 2015;**9**(11):11075-11089

[106] Jiao F, Hu H, Yuan C, Wang L, Jiang W, Jin Z, et al. Elevated expression level of long noncoding RNA MALAT-1 facilitates cell growth, migration and invasion in pancreatic cancer. Oncology Reports. 2014;**32**(6):2485-2492

[107] Jiao F, Hu H, Han T, Yuan C, Wang L, Jin Z, et al. Long noncoding RNA MALAT-1 enhances stem cell-like phenotypes in pancreatic cancer cells. International Journal of Molecular Sciences. 2015;**16**(4):6677-6693

[108] Cheng Y, Jutooru I, Chadalapaka G, Corton JC, Safe S. The long non-coding RNA HOTTIP enhances pancreatic cancer cell proliferation, survival and migration. Oncotarget. 2015;**6**(13):10840-10852

[109] Xie Z, Chen X, Li J, Guo Y, Li H, Pan X, et al. Salivary HOTAIR and PVT1 as novel biomarkers for early pancreatic cancer. Oncotarget. 2016;**7**(18):25408-25419

[110] Huang C, Yu W, Wang Q, Cui H, Wang Y, Zhang L, et al. Increased expression of the lncRNA PVT1 is associated with poor prognosis in pancreatic cancer patients. Minerva Medica. 2015;**106**(3):143-149

[111] Ma L, Tian X, Wang F, Zhang Z, Du C, Xie X, et al. The long noncoding RNA H19 promotes cell proliferation via E2F-1 in pancreatic ductal adenocarcinoma. Cancer Biology and Therapy. 2016;**17**(10):1051-1061

[112] Chen P, Wan D, Zheng D, Zheng Q, Wu F, Zhi Q. Long non-coding RNA UCA1 promotes the tumorigenesis in pancreatic cancer. Biomedicine & Pharmacotherapy. 2016;**83**:1220-1226

[113] Li Z, Zhao X, Zhou Y, Liu Y, Zhou Q, Ye H, et al. The long non-coding RNA HOTTIP promotes progression and gemcitabine resistance by regulating HOXA13 in pancreatic cancer. Journal of Translational Medicine. 2015;**13**:84

[114] Wang Y, Li Z, Zheng S, Zhou Y, Zhao L, Ye H, et al. Expression profile of long non-coding RNAs in pancreatic cancer and their clinical significance as biomarkers. Oncotarget. 2015;**6**(34):35684-35698

[115] Liu C, Wang J, Yuan X, Qian W, Zhang B, Shi M, et al. Long noncoding RNA uc.345 promotes tumorigenesis of pancreatic cancer by upregulation of hnRNPL expression. Oncotarget. 2016;**7**(44):71556-71566

[116] Lian Y, Wang J, Feng J, Ding J, Ma Z, Li J, et al. Long non-coding RNA IRAIN suppresses apoptosis and promotes proliferation by binding to LSD1 and EZH2 in pancreatic cancer. Tumour Biology. 2016;**37**(11):14929-14937

[117] Yin DD, Zhang EB, You LH, Wang N, Wang LT, Jin FY, et al. Downregulation of lncRNA TUG1 affects apoptosis and insulin secretion in mouse pancreatic β cells. Cellular Physiology and Biochemistry. 2015;**35**(5):1892-1904

[118] Peng W, Jiang A. Long noncoding RNA CCDC26 as a potential predictor biomarker contributes to tumorigenesis in pancreatic cancer. Biomedicine & Pharmacotherapy. 2016;**83**:712-717

[119] Zhan HX, Wang Y, Li C, Xu JW, Zhou B, Zhu JK, et al. LincRNA-ROR promotes invasion, metastasis and tumor growth in pancreatic cancer through activating ZEB1 pathway. Cancer Letters. 2016;**374**(2):261-271

[120] Li L, Zhang GQ, Chen H, Zhao ZJ, Chen HZ, Liu H, et al. Plasma and tumor levels of Linc-pint are diagnostic and prognostic biomarkers for pancreatic cancer. Oncotarget. 2016;**7**(44):71773-71781

[121] Sun XL, Cao GH, Cao Y, Jiang X, Li XK, Ye XH, et al. Association of LncRNA HMlincRNA717 with prognosis in pancreatic cancer. European Review for Medical and Pharmacological Sciences. 2016;**20**(11):2230-2234

[122] Zheng J, Huang X, Tan W, Yu D, Du Z, Chang J, et al. Pancreatic cancer risk variant in LINC00673 creates a miR-1231 binding site and interferes with PTPN11 degradation. Nature Genetics. 2016;**48**(7):747-757

[123] Fellenberg J, Bernd L, Delling G, Witte D, Zahlten-Hinguranage A. Prognostic significance of drug-regulated genes in high-grade osteosarcoma. Modern Pathology. 2007;**20**(10):1085-1094

[124] Ren YK, Xiao Y, Wan XB, Zhao YZ, Li J, Li Y, et al. Association of long non-coding RNA HOTTIP with progression and prognosis in colorectal cancer. International Journal of Clinical and Experimental Pathology. 2015;**8**(9):11458-11463

[125] Zhang H, Zhao L, Wang YX, Xi M, Liu SL, Luo LL. Long non-coding RNA HOTTIP is correlated with progression and prognosis in tongue squamous cell carcinoma. Tumour Biology. 2015;**36**(11):8805-8809

[126] Quagliata L, Matter MS, Piscuoglio S, Arabi L, Ruiz C, Procino A, et al. Long noncoding RNA HOTTIP/HOXA13 expression is associated with disease progression and predicts outcome in hepatocellular carcinoma patients. Hepatology. 2014;**59**(3):911-923

[127] Zheng X, Hu H, Li S. High expression of lncRNA PVT1 promotes invasion by inducing epithelial-to-mesenchymal transition in esophageal cancer. Oncology Letters. 2016;**12**(4):2357-2362

[128] Wan L, Sun M, Liu GJ, Wei CC, Zhang EB, Kong R, et al. Long noncoding RNA PVT1 promotes non-small cell lung cancer cell proliferation through epigenetically regulating LATS2 expression. Molecular Cancer Therapeutics. 2016;**15**(5):1082-1094

[129] Zeng C, Yu X, Lai J, Yang L, Chen S, Li Y. Overexpression of the long non-coding RNA PVT1 is correlated with leukemic cell proliferation in acute promyelocytic leukemia. Journal of Hematology & Oncology. 2015;**8**:126

[130] Zhuang C, Li J, Liu Y, Chen M, Yuan J, Fu X, et al. Tetracycline-inducible shRNA targeting long non-coding RNA PVT1 inhibits cell growth and induces apoptosis in bladder cancer cells. Oncotarget. 2015;**6**(38):41194-41203

[131] Kong R, Zhang EB, Yin DD, You LH, Xu TP, Chen WM, et al. Long noncoding RNA PVT1 indicates a poor prognosis of gastric cancer and promotes cell proliferation through epigenetically regulating p15 and p16. Molecular Cancer. 2015;**14**:82

[132] Yang YR, Zang SZ, Zhong CL, Li YX, Zhao SS, Feng XJ. Increased expression of the lncRNA PVT1 promotes tumorigenesis in non-small cell lung cancer. International Journal of Clinical and Experimental Pathology. 2014;**7**(10):6929-6935

[133] Zhang Z, Zhu Z, Zhang B, Li W, Li X, Wu X, et al. Frequent mutation of rs13281615 and its association with PVT1 expression and cell proliferation in breastcancer. Journal of Genetics and Genomics. 2014;**41**(4):187-195

[134] Zhang S, Zhang G, Liu J. Long noncoding RNA PVT1 promotes cervical cancer progression through epigenetically silencing miR-200b. APMIS. 2016;**124**(8):649-658

[135] Iden M, Fye S, Li K, Chowdhury T, Ramchandran R, Rader JS. The lncRNA PVT1 contributes to the cervical cancer phenotype and associates with poor patient prognosis. PLoS One. 2016;**11**(5):e0156274

[136] Yuan CL, Li H, Zhu L, Liu Z, Zhou J, Shu Y. Aberrant expression of long noncoding RNA PVT1 and its diagnostic and prognostic significance in patients with gastric cancer. Neoplasma. 2016;**63**(3):442-449

[137] Ding J, Li D, Gong M, Wang J, Huang X, Wu T, et al. Expression and clinical significance of the long non-coding RNA PVT1 in human gastric cancer. OncoTargets and Therapy. 2014;**7**:1625-1630

[138] Liu E, Liu Z, Zhou Y, Mi R, Wang D. Overexpression of long non-coding RNA PVT1 in ovarian cancer cells promotes cisplatin resistance by regulating apoptotic pathways. International Journal of Clinical and Experimental Medicine. 2015;**8**(11):20565-20572

[139] Zhang XW, Bu P, Liu L, Zhang XZ, Li J. Overexpression of long non-coding RNA PVT1 in gastric cancer cells promotes the development of multidrug resistance. Biochemical and Biophysical Research Communications. 2015;**462**(3):227-232

[140] Zhou Q, Chen J, Feng J, Wang J. Long noncoding RNA PVT1 modulates thyroid cancer cell proliferation by recruiting EZH2 and regulating thyroid-stimulating hormone receptor (TSHR). Tumour Biology. 2016;**37**(3):3105-3113

[141] Takahashi Y, Sawada G, Kurashige J, Uchi R, Matsumura T, Ueo H, et al. Amplification of PVT-1 is involved in poor prognosis via apoptosis inhibition in colorectal cancers. British Journal of Cancer. 2014;**110**(1):164-171

[142] Yang JP, Yang XJ, Xiao L, Wang Y. Long noncoding RNA PVT1 as a novel serum biomarker for detection of cervical cancer. European Review for Medical and Pharmacological Sciences. 2016;**20**(19):3980-3986

[143] Yu J, Han J, Zhang J, Li G, Liu H, Cui X, et al. The long noncoding RNAs PVT1 and uc002mbe.2 in sera provide a new supplementary method for hepatocellular carcinoma diagnosis. Medicine (Baltimore). 2016;**95**(31):e4436

[144] Wu Y, Wang YQ, Weng WW, Zhang QY, Yang XQ, Gan HL, et al. A serum-circulating long noncoding RNA signature can discriminate between patients with clear cell renal cell carcinoma and healthy controls. Oncogenesis. 2016;**5**:e192

[145] Ding C, Yang Z, Lv Z, Du C, Xiao H, Peng C, et al. Long non-coding RNA PVT1 is associated with tumor progression and predicts recurrence in hepatocellular carcinoma patients. Oncology Letters. 2015;**9**(2):955-963

[146] Ding C, Cheng S, Yang Z, Lv Z, Xiao H, Du C, et al. Long non-coding RNA HOTAIR promotes cell migration and invasion via down-regulation of RNA binding motif protein 38 in hepatocellular carcinoma cells. International Journal of Molecular Sciences. 2014;**15**(3):4060-4076

[147] Lee M, Kim HJ, Kim SW, Park SA, Chun KH, Cho NH, et al. The long non-coding RNA HOTAIR increases tumour growth and invasion in cervical cancer by targeting the Notch pathway. Oncotarget. 2016;**7**(28):44558-44571

[148] Luo ZF, Zhao D, Li XQ, Cui YX, Ma N, Lu CX, et al. Clinical significance of HOTAIR expression in colon cancer. World Journal of Gastroenterology. 2016;**22**(22):5254-5259

[149] Sun W, Yang Y, Xu C, Xie Y, Guo J. Roles of long noncoding RNAs in gastric cancer and their clinical applications. Journal of Cancer Research and Clinical Oncology. 2016;**142**(11):2231-2237

[150] Dong L, Hui L. HOTAIR promotes proliferation, migration, and invasion of ovarian cancer SKOV3 cells through regulating PIK3R3. Medical Science Monitor. 2016;**22**:325-331

[151] Zhu Y, Yu RK, Ji AF, Yao XL, Fang JJ, Jin XD. Effects of long non-coding RNA-HOTAIR on the cell cycle and invasiveness of prostate cancer. [Article in Chinese] Zhonghua Nan Ke Xue. 2015;**21**(9):792-796

[152] Yang XD, Xu HT, Xu XH, Ru G, Liu W, Zhu JJ, et al. Knockdown of long non-coding RNA HOTAIR inhibits proliferation and invasiveness and improves radiosensitivity in colorectal cancer. Oncology Reports. 2016;**35**(1):479-487

[153] Li H, An J, Wu M, Zheng Q, Gui X, Li T, et al. LncRNA HOTAIR promotes human liver cancer stem cell malignant growth through downregulation of SETD2. Oncotarget. 2015;**6**(29):27847-27864

[154] Yiwei T, Hua H, Hui G, Mao M, Xiang L. HOTAIR interacting with MAPK1 regulates ovarian cancer skov3 cell proliferation, migration, and invasion. Medical Science Monitor. 2015;**21**:1856-1863

[155] Zhou C, Ye L, Jiang C, Bai J, Chi Y, Zhang H. Long noncoding RNA HOTAIR, a hypoxiainducible factor-1α activated driver of malignancy, enhances hypoxic cancer cell proliferation, migration, and invasion in non-small cell lung cancer. Tumour Biology. 2015;**36**(12):9179-9188

[156] Milevskiy MJ, Al-Ejeh F, Saunus JM, Northwood KS, Bailey PJ, Betts JA, et al. Longrange regulators of the lncRNA HOTAIR enhance its prognostic potential in breast cancer. Human Molecular Genetics. 2016;**25**(15):3269-3283

[157] Qiu H, Liu Q, Li J, Wang X, Wang Y, Yuan Z, et al. Analysis of the association of HOTAIR single nucleotide polymorphism (rs920778) and risk of cervical cancer. APMIS. 2016;**124**(7):567-573

[158] Gao JZ, Li J, Du JL, Li XL. Long non-coding RNA HOTAIR is a marker for hepatocellular carcinoma progression and tumor recurrence. Oncology Letters. 2016;**11**(3):1791-1798

[159] Berrondo C, Flax J, Kucherov V, Siebert A, Osinski T, Rosenberg A, et al. Expression of the long non-coding RNA HOTAIR correlates with disease progression in bladder cancer and is contained in bladder cancer patient urinary exosomes. PLoS One. 2016;**11**(1):e0147236

[160] Shang C, Guo Y, Zhang H, Xue YX. Long noncoding RNA HOTAIR is a prognostic biomarker and inhibits chemosensitivity to doxorubicin in bladder transitional cell carcinoma. Cancer Chemotherapy and Pharmacology. 2016;**77**(3):507-513

[161] Xue X, Yang YA, Zhang A, Fong KW, Kim J, Song B, et al. LncRNA HOTAIR enhances ER signaling and confers tamoxifen resistance in breast cancer. Oncogene. 2016;**35**(21):2746-2755

[162] Li J, Yang S, Su N, Wang Y, Yu J, Qiu H, et al. Overexpression of long non-coding RNA HOTAIR leads to chemoresistance by activating the Wnt/β-catenin pathway in human ovarian cancer. Tumour Biology. 2016;**37**(2):2057-2065

[163] Wu H, Shang X, Shi Y, Yang Z, Zhao J, Yang M, et al. Genetic variants of lncRNA HOTAIR and risk of epithelial ovarian cancer among Chinese women. Oncotarget. 2016;**7**(27):41047-41052

[164] Dou J, Ni Y, He X, Wu D, Li M, Wu S, et al. Decreasing lncRNA HOTAIR expression inhibits human colorectal cancer stem cells. American Journal of Translational Research. 2016;**8**(1):98-108

[165] Yang L, Zhang X, Li H, Liu J. The long noncoding RNA HOTAIR activates autophagy by upregulating ATG3 and ATG7 in hepatocellular carcinoma. Molecular Biosystems. 2016;12(8):2605-2612

[166] Sun J, Chu H, Ji J, Huo G, Song Q, Zhang X. Long non-coding RNA HOTAIR modulates HLA-G expression by absorbing miR-148a in human cervical cancer. International Journal of Oncology. 2016;**49**(3):943-952

[167] Song B, Guan Z, Liu F, Sun D, Wang K, Qu H. Long non-coding RNA HOTAIR promotes HLA-G expression via inhibiting miR-152 in gastric cancer cells. Biochemical and Biophysical Research Communications. 2015;**464**(3):807-813

[168] Kishikawa T, Otsuka M, Ohno M, Yoshikawa T, Takata A, Koike K. Circulating RNAs as new biomarkers for detecting pancreatic cancer. World Journal of Gastroenterology. 2015;**21**(28):8527-8540

[169] Zhang Y, Zhang K, Luo Z, Liu L, Wu L, Liu J. Circulating long non-coding HOX transcript antisense intergenic ribonucleic acid in plasma as a potential biomarker for diagnosis of breast cancer. Thoracic Cancer. 2016;**7**(6):627-632

[170] Zhao W, Song M, Zhang J, Kuerban M, Wang H. Combined identification of long non-coding RNA CCAT1 and HOTAIR in serum as an effective screening for colorectal carcinoma. International Journal of Clinical and Experimental Pathology. 2015;**8**(11):14131-14140

[171] Arita T, Ichikawa D, Konishi H, Komatsu S, Shiozaki A, Shoda K, et al. Circulating long non-coding RNAs in plasma of patients with gastric cancer. Anticancer Research. 2013;**33**(8):3185-3193

[172] Wang L, Sun Y, Yi J, Wang X, Liang J, Pan Z, et al. Targeting H19 by lentivirus-mediated RNA interference increases A549 cell migration and invasion. Experimental Lung Research. 2016;**42**(7):346-353

[173] Jiang X, Yan Y, Hu M, Chen X, Wang Y, Dai Y, et al. Increased level of H19 long noncoding RNA promotes invasion, angiogenesis, and stemness of glioblastoma cells. Journal of Neurosurgery. 2016;**124**(1):129-136

[174] Berteaux N, Lottin S, Monté D, Pinte S, Quatannens B, Coll J, et al. H19 mRNA-like noncoding RNA promotes breast cancer cell proliferation through positive control by E2F1. The Journal of Biological Chemistry. 2005;**280**(33):29625-29636

[175] Jing W, Zhu M, Zhang XW, Pan ZY, Gao SS, Zhou H, et al. The significance of long noncoding RNA H19 in predicting progression and metastasis of cancers: A meta-analysis. BioMed Research International. 2016;**2016**:5902678

[176] Wang SH, Wu XC, Zhang MD, Weng MZ, Zhou D, Quan ZW. Upregulation of H19 indicates a poor prognosis in gallbladder carcinoma and promotes epithelial-mesenchymal transition. American Journal of Cancer Research. 2015;**6**(1):15-26

[177] Han D, Gao X, Wang M, Qiao Y, Xu Y, Yang J, et al. Long noncoding RNA H19 indicates a poor prognosis of colorectal cancer and promotes tumor growth by recruiting and binding to eIF4A3. Oncotarget. 2016;**7**(16):22159-22173

[178] Wang SH, Wu XC, Zhang MD, Weng MZ, Zhou D, Quan ZW. Long noncoding RNA H19 contributes to gallbladder cancer cell proliferation by modulated miR-194-5p targeting AKT2. Tumour Biology. 2016;**37**(7):9721-9730

[179] Zhang E, Li W, Yin D, De W, Zhu L, Sun S, et al. c-Myc-regulated long non-coding RNA H19 indicates a poor prognosis and affects cell proliferation in non-small-cell lung cancer. Tumour Biology. 2016;**37**(3):4007-4015

[180] Jia P, Cai H, Liu X, Chen J, Ma J, Wang P, et al. Long non-coding RNA H19 regulates glioma angiogenesis and the biological behavior of glioma-associated endothelial cells by inhibiting microRNA-29a. Cancer Letters. 2016;**381**(2):359-369

[181] Zheng ZG, Xu H, Suo SS, Xu XL, Ni MW, Gu LH, et al. The essential role of H19 contributing to cisplatin resistance by regulating glutathione metabolism in high-grade serous ovarian cancer. Scientific Reports. 2016;**6**:26093

[182] Li W, Jiang P, Sun X, Xu S, Ma X, Zhan R. Suppressing H19 modulates tumorigenicity and stemness in U251 and U87MG glioma cells. Cellular and Molecular Neurobiology.2016;**36**(8):1219-1227

[183] Zeira E, Abramovitch R, Meir K, Even Ram S, Gil Y, Bulvik B, et al. The knockdown of H19lncRNA reveals its regulatory role in pluripotency and tumorigenesis of human embryonic carcinoma cells. Oncotarget. 2015;**6**(33):34691-34703

[184] Huang C, Cao L, Qiu L, Dai X, Ma L, Zhou Y, et al. Upregulation of H19 promotes invasion and induces epithelial-to-mesenchymal transition in esophageal cancer. Oncology Letters. 2015;**10**(1):291-296

[185] Liang WC, Fu WM, Wong CW, Wang Y, Wang WM, Hu GX, et al. The lncRNA H19 promotes epithelial to mesenchymal transition by functioning as miRNA sponges in colorectal cancer. Oncotarget. 2015;**6**(26):22513-22525

[186] Hidalgo M, Cascinu S, Kleeff J, Labianca R, Löhr JM, Neoptolemos J, et al. Addressing the challenges of pancreatic cancer: Future directions for improving outcomes. Pancreatology. 2013;**15**(1):8-18

[187] Yang T, Zeng H, Chen W, Zheng R, Zhang Y, Li Z, et al. Helicobacter pylori infection, H19 and LINC00152 expression in serum and risk of gastric cancer in a Chinese population. Cancer Epidemiology. 2016;**44**:147-153

[188] Hua Q, Lv X, Gu X, Chen Y, Chu H, Du M, et al. Genetic variants in lncRNA H19 are associated with the risk of bladder cancer in a Chinese population. Mutagenesis. 2016;**31**(5):531-538

[189] Feng J, Sun Y, Zhang EB, Lu XY, Jin SD, Guo RH. A novel long noncoding RNA IRAIN regulates cell proliferation in nonsmall cell lung cancer. International Journal of Clinical and Experimental Pathology. 2015;**8**(10):12268-12275

[190] Kang L, Sun J, Wen X, Cui J, Wang G, Hoffman AR, et al. Aberrant allele-switch imprinting of a novel IGF1R intragenic antisense non-coding RNA in breast cancers. European. Journal of Cancer. 2015;**51**(2):260-270

[191] Lu L, Shen Y, Tseng KF, Liu W, Duan H, Meng W. Silencing of UCA1, a poor prognostic factor, inhibited the migration of endometrial cancer cell. Cancer Biomarkers. 2016;**17**(2):171-177

[192] Bian Z, Jin L, Zhang J, Yin Y, Quan C, Hu Y, et al. LncRNA-UCA1 enhances cell proliferation and 5-fluorouracil resistance in colorectal cancer by inhibiting miR-204-5p. Scientific Reports. 2016;6:23892

[193] Nie W, Ge HJ, Yang XQ, Sun X, Huang H, Tao X, et al. LncRNA-UCA1 exerts oncogenic functions in non-small cell lung cancer by targeting miR-193a-3p. Cancer Letters. 2016;**371**(1):99-106

[194] Na XY, Liu ZY, Ren PP, Yu R, Shang XS. Long non-coding RNA UCA1 contributes to the progression of prostate cancer and regulates proliferation through KLF4-KRT6/13 signaling pathway. International Journal of Clinical and Experimental Medicine. 2015;**8**(8):12609-12616

[195] Yang YT, Wang YF, Lai JY, Shen SY, Wang F, Kong J, et al. Long non-coding RNA UCA1 contributes to the progression of oral squamous cell carcinoma via regulating WNT/β-catenin signaling pathway. Cancer Science. 2016;**107**(11):1581-1589

[196] Li JY, Ma X, Zhang CB. Overexpression of long non-coding RNA UCA1 predicts a poor prognosis in patients with esophageal squamous cell carcinoma. International Journal of Clinical and Experimental Pathology. 2014;**7**(11):7938-7944

[197] Xiao C, Wu CH, Hu HZ. LncRNA UCA1 promotes epithelial-mesenchymal transition (EMT) of breast cancer cells via enhancing Wnt/beta-catenin signaling pathway. European Review for Medical and Pharmacological Sciences. 2016;**20**(13):2819-2824

[198] Yang Y, Jiang Y, Wan Y, Zhang L, Qiu J, Zhou S, et al. UCA1 functions as a competing endogenous RNA to suppress epithelial ovarian cancer metastasis. Tumour Biology. 2016;**37**(8):10633-10641

[199] Lee JJ, Kim M, Kim HP. Epigenetic regulation of long noncoding RNA UCA1 by SATB1 in breast cancer. BMB Reports. 2016;**49**(10):578-583

[200] Tuo YL, Li XM, Luo J. Long noncoding RNA UCA1 modulates breast cancer cell growth and apoptosis through decreasing tumor suppressive miR-143. European Review for Medical and Pharmacological Sciences. 2015;**19**(18):3403-3411

[201] Wang X, Yang B, Ma B. The UCA1/miR-204/Sirt1 axis modulates docetaxel sensitivity of prostate cancer cells. Cancer Chemotherapy and Pharmacology. 2016;**78**(5):1025-1031

[202] Wu C, Luo J. Long non-coding RNA (lncRNA) urothelial carcinoma-associated 1 (UCA1) enhances tamoxifen resistance in breast cancer cells via inhibiting mTOR signaling pathway. Medical Science Monitor. 2016;**22**:3860-3867

[203] Pan J, Li X, Wu W, Xue M, Hou H, Zhai W. Long non-coding RNA UCA1 promotes cisplatin/gemcitabine resistance through CREB modulating miR-196a-5p in bladder cancer cells. Cancer Letters. 2016;**382**(1):64-76

[204] Fang Q, Chen X, Zhi X. Long non-coding RNA (LncRNA) urothelial carcinoma associated 1 (UCA1) increases multi-drug resistance of gastric cancer via downregulating miR-27b. Medical Science Monitor. 2016;**22**:3506-3513

[205] Li X, Wu Y, Liu A, Tang X. Long non-coding RNA UCA1 enhances tamoxifen resistance in breast cancer cells through a miR-18a-HIF1α feedback regulatory loop. Tumour Biology. 2016;**37**(11):14733-14743

[206] Li HJ, Li X, Pang H, Pan JJ, Xie XJ, Chen W. Long non-coding RNA UCA1 promotes glutamine metabolism by targeting miR-16 in human bladder cancer. Japanese Journal of Clinical Oncology. 2015;**45**(11):1055-1063

[207] Hariharan D, Saied A, Kocher HM. Analysis of mortality rates for pancreatic cancer across the world. HPB. 2008;**10**(1):58-62

[208] El-Tawdi AH, Matboli M, El-Nakeep S, Azazy AE, Abdel-Rahman O. Association of long noncoding RNA and c-JUN expression in hepatocellular carcinoma. Expert Review of Gastroenterology & Hepatology. 2016;**10**(7):869-877

[209] Gao J, Cao R, Mu H. Long non-coding RNA UCA1 may be a novel diagnostic and predictive biomarker in plasma for early gastric cancer.

[210] Tao K, Yang J, Hu Y, Sun Y, Tan Z, Duan J, et al. Clinical significance of urothelial carcinoma associated 1 in colon cancer. International Journal of Clinical and Experimental Medicine. 2015;**8**(11):21854-21860

[211] Wang HM, Lu JH, Chen WY, Gu AQ. Upregulated lncRNA-UCA1 contributes to progression of lung cancer and is closely related to clinical diagnosis as a predictive biomarker in plasma. International Journal of Clinical and Experimental Medicine. 2015;**8**(7):11824-11830

[212] Milowich D, Le Mercier M, De Neve N, Sandras F, Roumeguere T, Decaestecker C, et al. Diagnostic value of the UCA1 test for bladder cancer detection: A clinical study. Springerplus. 2015;**4**:349

[213] Eissa S, Matboli M, Essawy NO, Shehta M, Kotb YM. Rapid detection of urinary long non-coding RNA urothelial carcinoma associated one using a PCR-free nanoparticle-based assay. Biomarkers. 2015;**20**(3):212-217

[214] Eissa S, Matboli M, Essawy NO, Kotb YM. Integrative functional genetic-epigenetic approach for selecting genes as urine biomarkers for bladder cancer diagnosis. Tumour Biology. 2015;**36**(12):9545-9552

[215] Srivastava AK, Singh PK, Rath SK, Dalela D, Goel MM, Bhatt ML. Appraisal of diagnostic ability of UCA1 as a biomarker of carcinoma of the urinary bladder. Tumour Biology. 2014;**35**(11):11435-11442

[216] Zhang Z, Hao H, Zhang CJ, Yang XY, He Q, Lin J. Evaluation of novel gene UCA1 as a tumor biomarker for the detection of bladder cancer. [Article in Chinese] Zhonghua Yi Xue Za Zhi. 2012;**92**(6):384-387

[217] Wang XS, Zhang Z, Wang HC, Cai JL, Xu QW, Li MQ, et al. Rapid identification of UCA1 as a very sensitive and specific unique marker for human bladder carcinoma. Clinical Cancer Research. 2006;**12**(16):4851-4858

[218] Zhao XB, Ren GS. WITHDRAWN: LncRNA TUG1 promotes breast cancer cell proliferation via inhibiting miR-9. Cancer Biomarkers. 2016. DOI: 10.3233/CBM-160669

[219] Iliev R, Kleinova R, Juracek J, Dolezel J, Ozanova Z, Fedorko M, et al. Overexpression of long non-coding RNA TUG1 predicts poor prognosis and promotes cancer cell proliferation and migration in high-grade muscle-invasive bladder cancer. Tumour Biology. 2016;**37**(10):13385-13390

[220] Huang MD, Chen WM, Qi FZ, Sun M, Xu TP, Ma P, et al. Long non-coding RNA TUG1 is up-regulated in hepatocellular carcinoma and promotes cell growth and apoptosis by epigenetically silencing of KLF2. Molecular Cancer. 2015;**14**:165

[221] Xu Y, Wang J, Qiu M, Xu L, Li M, Jiang F, et al. Upregulation of the long noncoding RNA TUG1 promotes proliferation and migration of esophageal squamous cell carcinoma. Tumour Biology. 2015;**36**(3):1643-1651

[222] Zhang Q, Geng PL, Yin P, Wang XL, Jia JP, Yao J. Down-regulation of long non-coding RNA TUG1 inhibits osteosarcoma cell proliferation and promotes apoptosis. Asian Pacific Journal of Cancer Prevention. 2013;**14**(4):2311-2315

[223] Kuang D, Zhang X, Hua S, Dong W, Li Z. Long non-coding RNA TUG1 regulates ovarian cancer proliferation and metastasis via affecting epithelial-mesenchymal transition. Experimental and Molecular Pathology. 2016;**101**(2):267-273

[224] Zhai HY, Sui MH, Yu X, Qu Z, Hu JC, Sun HQ, et al. Overexpression of long non-coding RNA TUG1 promotes colon cancer progression. Medical Science Monitor. 2016;**22**:3281-3287

[225] Zhang E, He X, Yin D, Han L, Qiu M, Xu T, et al. Increased expression of long noncoding RNA TUG1 predicts a poor prognosis of gastric cancer and regulates cell proliferation by epigenetically silencing of p57. Cell Death & Disease. 2016;**7**:e2109

[226] Sun J, Ding C, Yang Z, Liu T, Zhang X, Zhao C, et al. The long non-coding RNA TUG1 indicates a poor prognosis for colorectal cancer and promotes metastasis by affecting epithelial-mesenchymal transition. Journal of Translational Medicine. 2016;**14**:42

[227] Jiang L, Wang W, Li G, Sun C, Ren Z, Sheng H, et al. High TUG1 expression is associated with chemotherapy resistance and poor prognosis in esophageal squamous cell carcinoma. Cancer Chemotherapy and Pharmacology. 2016;**78**(2):333-339

[228] Li J, Zhang M, An G, Ma Q. LncRNA TUG1 acts as a tumor suppressor in human glioma by promoting cell apoptosis. Experimental Biology and Medicine (Maywood, N.J.). 2016;**241**(6):644-649

[229] Ma B, Li M, Zhang L, Huang M, Lei JB, Fu GH, et al. Upregulation of long non-coding RNA TUG1 correlates with poor Tumour Biology. 2016;**37**(4):4445-4455

[230] Isin M, Ozgur E, Cetin G, Erten N, Aktan M, Gezer U, et al. Investigation of circulating lncRNAs in B-cell neoplasms. Clinica Chimica Acta. 2014;**431**:255-259

Chapter 2

Exploiting Exosomes for Differential Diagnosis of Multiple Myeloma and Monoclonal Gammopathy of Undetermined Significance

Lucia Paolini, Giuseppe Di Noto, Andrea Zendrini,
Paolo Bergese and Doris Ricotta

Additional information is available at the end of the chapter

http://dx.doi.org/10.5772/intechopen.69398

Abstract

Multiple myeloma (MM) is a plasma cell dyscrasia characterized by a clonal plasma cell proliferation. Usually, all MM are preceded by an asymptomatic premalignant stage termed monoclonal gammopathy of undetermined significance (MGUS). Differential diagnosis requires the evidence of end-organ damage, but recently new biomarkers are emerging to help clinicians to distinguish MM from the premalignant phase. Circulating exosomes in serum seem to be a powerful tool to be analyzed for liquid biopsy, and in this chapter, we show that MM and MGUS exosomes are different in concentration, biological activity, and biochemical markers. These differences seem to be related to the free light chains (FLCs) associated with exosomes and their propathogenic properties. The cellular processing FLC-decorated exosomes and their ability to activate proinflammatory mechanisms are different in MM and MGUS patients. These elements can be evaluated to create an innovative multiparameter panel to monitor MGUS to MM switching.

Keywords: multiple myeloma, exosomes, biomarkers, MGUS

1. Introduction

This chapter aims to show the possibility of differential typization of multiple myeloma (MM) and monoclonal gammopathy of undetermined significance (MGUS) serum-derived exosomes exploiting an innovative biochemical and bio-physical approach, in order to evaluate new biomarkers for the differential diagnosis among these two conditions.

MM is a plasma cell dyscrasia characterized by a clonal plasma cell proliferation. The worldwide MM incidence is 3.29/100,000 and increases with age. In the 80–84 years old population, the rate is 37.1, while the median age of diagnosis is 73 years [1]. Usually, almost all MM are preceded by an asymptomatic premalignant stage termed MGUS [2]. MGUS is present in roughly 3–4% of the population over the age of 50 years and it is associated with a risk of progression to MM of approximately 1% [3]. MGUS is clinically silent and is usually diagnosed incidentally when a monoclonal (M) protein is detected during laboratory work-up of patients who have a wide spectrum of clinical conditions. The diagnosis of MGUS requires the absence of hypercalcemia, renal failure, anemia, and bone lesions (CRAB features) that can be attributed to the underlying plasma cell disorder.

Thus, over the years, the diagnosis of MM instead required evidence of end-organ damage attributable to the neoplastic clone of plasma cells in order to prevent MGUS patients from unnecessary and toxic chemotherapy. Furthermore, the MM diagnosis requires bone marrow examination like osteo-medullary biopsy to prove the presence of clonal bone marrow plasma cells [3]. Identification of new biomarkers of malignancy is fundamental to prevent end-organ damage in selected patients who are at imminent risk of symptomatic progression.

In this scenario, liquid biopsy could provide an alternative to invasive procedure and improve screening and early detection of cancer [4]. Liquid biopsy is defined as the search of biomarkers [5] in peripheral blood, and in recent years, exosomes have arisen as a powerful tool to understand cancer biology. Exosomes are vesicles with a size of 50–150 nm, which are secreted by cells into the extracellular space and play an important role in cell communication as cargoes of several specific proteins and RNAs. Exosomes are to date considered playing a pivotal role in information transfer in hematological malignancies [6] and recent studies show that specific exosomal microRNAs are involved in pathogenesis and have a prognostic role in MM [7]. In this chapter, we will analyze the biochemical and biological characteristics of MM and MGUS FLC and their cellular processing through exosomes. We show that free light chain (FLC)-decorated exosomes from patients carry peculiar bio-physical and biological qualities that allow the distinction of the malignant and premalignant condition.

2. MM and MGUS FLC cellular processing

In this section, we describe the potential pathogenic properties of serum FLC from MM and MGUS patients, correlating them with exosomal mediated cell-to-cell communication. About 80% of MM originates from intact immunoglobulin, non-IgM, MGUS and 20% from light-chain immunoglobulin MGUS [2]. Since 2009, the FLC quantitative assay (developed from both the Binding Site and Siemens) has been recommended by the International Myeloma Working Group to predict risk of progression in MGUS, the evaluation and management of MM [8]. This immunonephelometric assay allows the quantification of the kappa and lambda light chains untied to the heavy chains in serum [2, 9]. Calculation of the related kappa/lambda FLC ratio is an important parameter because about a third of patients with MGUS and more than 90% of patients with MM have altered FLC ratios that indicate excess production of a clonal FLC by the proliferating plasma cell population [2].

Thus, MGUS and MM patients can show similar serum FLC concentration with comparable FLC kappa/lambda ratio and the presence of FLC in urine is often confirmed by urine immunofixation [10]. Kappa and lambda FLCs have been long-considered a by-product of plasma cells, but evidences show that they possess intrinsic pathogenic characteristics [10] as in the case of AL amyloidosis, light-chain deposition disease, MM, and altered FLC ratio is associated with higher risk of progression in MGUS.

FLCs are able to disrupt the normal physiology of different organs, such as heart, kidney, and lungs. They are occasionally responsible for severe organ damage [11], and these multiple effects are probably related to their primary sequence or posttranslational modification [12] that can alter their biochemical properties, giving them particular affinity for some tissues with respect to others or activating different turnovers inside the cells [10]. This is confirmed for FLC present in serum of patients with MM and MGUS conditions: experiment *in vitro* showed different FLC internalization rate in endothelial, myocardial, and epithelia cell lines for the MM and MGUS FLC. Considering that FLCs circulate in the blood stream and that they interact with the vascular bed to reach the target tissue, Human Vein Endothelial Cells (HVEC), Rat heart myoblast (H9C2), and Human epithelioid cervix carcinoma (HeLa) cell lines are good models for organs usually involved in FLC tissue damage, respectively, for the endothelial, cardiac, and epithelial compartment. In Di Noto et al. [10], cells were incubated with serum of MM and MGUS patients at constant FLC concentration and results showed a faster internalization rate of MM FLC (after 1 h up to 16 h) compared with MGUS FLC in HeLa, HVEC, and H9C2, respectively (**Figure 1**). This suggests that cells are able to uptake FLC from the extracellular environment and FLCs from MM and MGUS patients have different affinity to these cell types even though all of them can be internalized after 16 h of exposure. In contrast, serum from healthy patients, without altered FLC values and kappa/lambda ratio did not show any similar properties probably because it did not contain FLC with propathological characteristics.

Considering these data, we could hypothesize that the interaction of FLC with peripheral districts depends on high-specific receptors expressed on certain cellular lines and/or that each patient has an individual clinical pattern due to the paraprotein molecular structure: thus, the differences between MM and MGUS can be related to peculiar FLC properties that can also alter their processing inside the cells [13].

It has been shown that FLC from AL amyloidosis patients induces oxidative stress and FLC internalization in cardiac fibroblasts enhances sulfatation of secreted glycosaminoglycans (GAGs) suggesting that the intracellular trafficking pathway of FLC could be correlated with the amyloidogenic potential of paraproteins [14]. Differences in FLC from MM and MGUS patients are not limited at the interaction with different cell type, but also their processing inside the cell is diverse: after intracellular internalization, they are rerouted in the extracellular melieu in different form, soluble or via pelletable extracellular vesicles (EVs).

HVEC and H9C2 cells were incubated for 4 h with serum from MM or MGUS patients containing a final FLC concentration of 20 μg/mL. After this initial step, cells were treated with trypsin, an enzyme able to cleave peptide chains, in order to eliminate FLC remained attached at the cell surface. Cells were, then, left in fresh medium (without FLC). After 16 h, the medium was collected

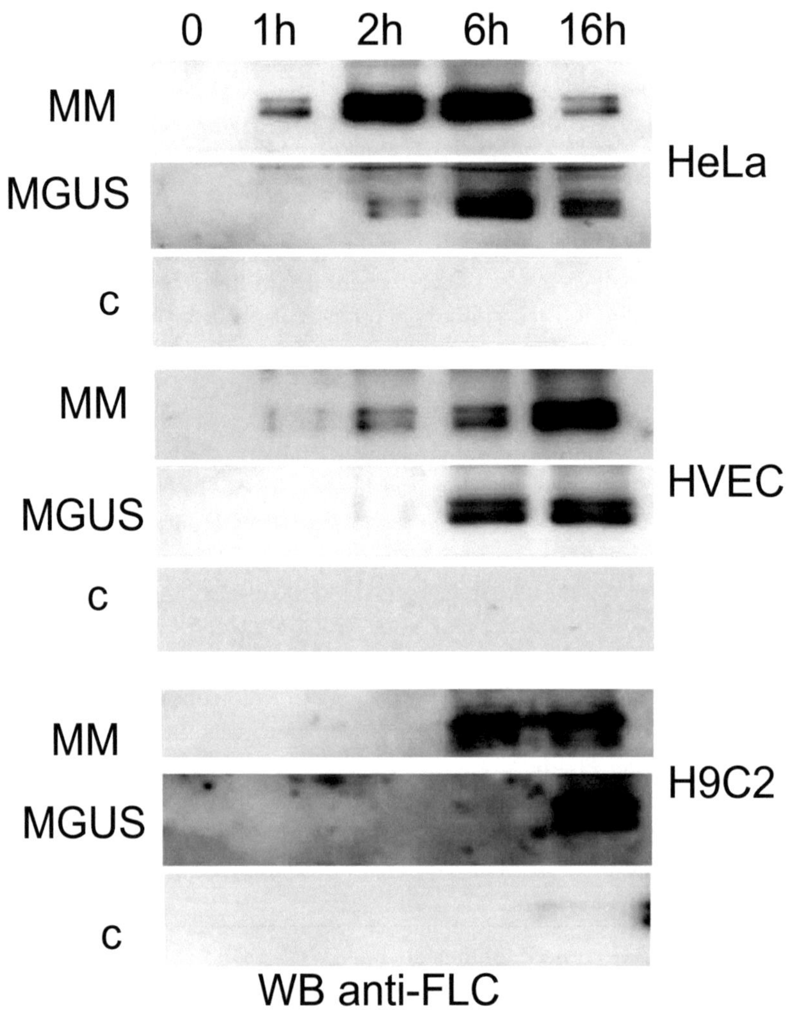

Figure 1. FLCs intracellular uptake. HeLa, HVEC, and H9C2 cell lines were incubated with serum of MM, MGUS at a final FLC concentration of 20 μg/mL and healthy donor (c). After incubation for 0, 1, 2, 6, and 16h cells were processed and analyzed by Western blot with anti-FLC antibody. Adapted from Di Noto et al. [10].

and submitted to a "three step centrifugation" protocol (800 × g 30 min, 16,000 × g 45 min, and 100,000 × g 2 h). This protocol allows the separation of different elements in biological fluids based on their size and density [15], exploiting the gravity force: the first centrifuge allowed to pellet cell debris and large vesicles like apoptotic bodies (P1), the second (P2) microvesicles budded from the plasma membrane (also called ectosomes, with diameters from 150 to 500 nm), while the ultracentrifugation step (P3) pellets smaller extracellular vesicles, like exosomes (50–150 nm) released through multivesicular bodies (MVBs) in the endosomal pathway [15]. FLCs from MM are internalized in cells after 4 h and subsequently released in the medium after 16 h (present in the P3), while MGUS FLCs are only present in cellular homogenate and in the third centrifuge super-

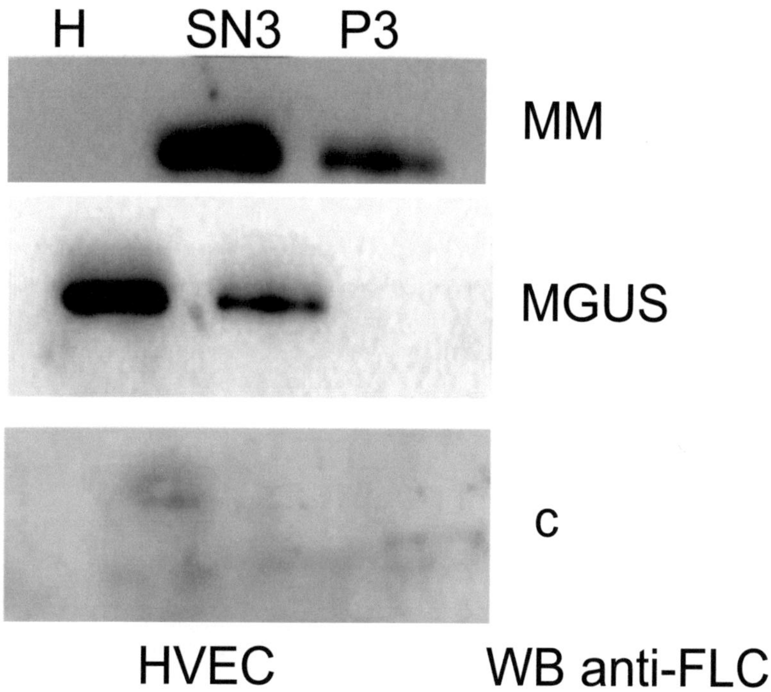

Figure 2. Extracellular rerouting of internalized FLC. HVEC cells were treated as described in the text. H: Homogenate, SN3: supernatant after 100,000 × g centrifugation, P3: pellet after 100,000 × g centrifugation. WB with antibodies anti-FLC. Adapted from Di Noto et al. [10].

natant (SN3). Cell incubated with healthy serum (c) did not give any signal as expected (**Figure 2**). Thus, the MM FLCs, after being internalized, are processed by the cells in a different way than MGUS and released outside the cell in vesicles that are pelleted at 100,000 × g, probably exosomes.

2.1. EVs from cell biochemical characterization

One of the criteria to characterize a population of vesicles and determine their nature is the immunoblot analysis or Western blot (WB) [16, 17]. According to the guidelines, it is important to show that at least three of the common exosomal markers are present in the sample. These protein lists are continuously updating and they include protein involved in exosomes formation (Alix, Hsp70, Annexin V, and Annexin XI), protein enriched in exosomes (tetraspanin CD63, CD81, CD9, and ADAM10) and from the endosomal compartment (TSG101, Syntenin-1, and VPS4B). WB analysis should also include negative controls: signal of protein is not enriched in exosomes (i.e., GM130 for the Cis-Golgi network, Calnexin for the endoplasmic reticulum) to verify the preparation purity from non-endosomal origin membrane. Especially for EVs deriving from cells, it is important to compare on the same gel identical amounts of protein from exosomes and from total lysates prepared from the producing cells to show an enrichment of the markers [16, 18]. In this scenario, Di Noto et al. [10]

showed the presence of the exosomal markers Annexin V, Hsp70, Caveolin 1, Lamp 1, and Tubulin in P3 derived from HVEC and H9C2 culture medium, after MM FLC internalization (**Figure 3**). We observed a Caveolin 1 positive signal in P3 of MGUS treated cells loading four times the amount of MM treated cells. Thus, the P3 preparation from cells contains exosomes and according to the semiquantitative analysis, with different amount from cells exposed to MM or MGUS serum.

It is important to highlight that in this study, Di Noto et al. analyzed the presence of the c-src protein in the cell-derived exosomes. C-src is a tyrosin kinase linked with inflammatory environment and osteolytic bone disease in MM [19] and Di Noto et al. [10] could show that the kinase was present only in exosomes generated during malignant FLC processing, while non-malignant FLCs are unable to induce c-src exosomal recruitment. This is the first

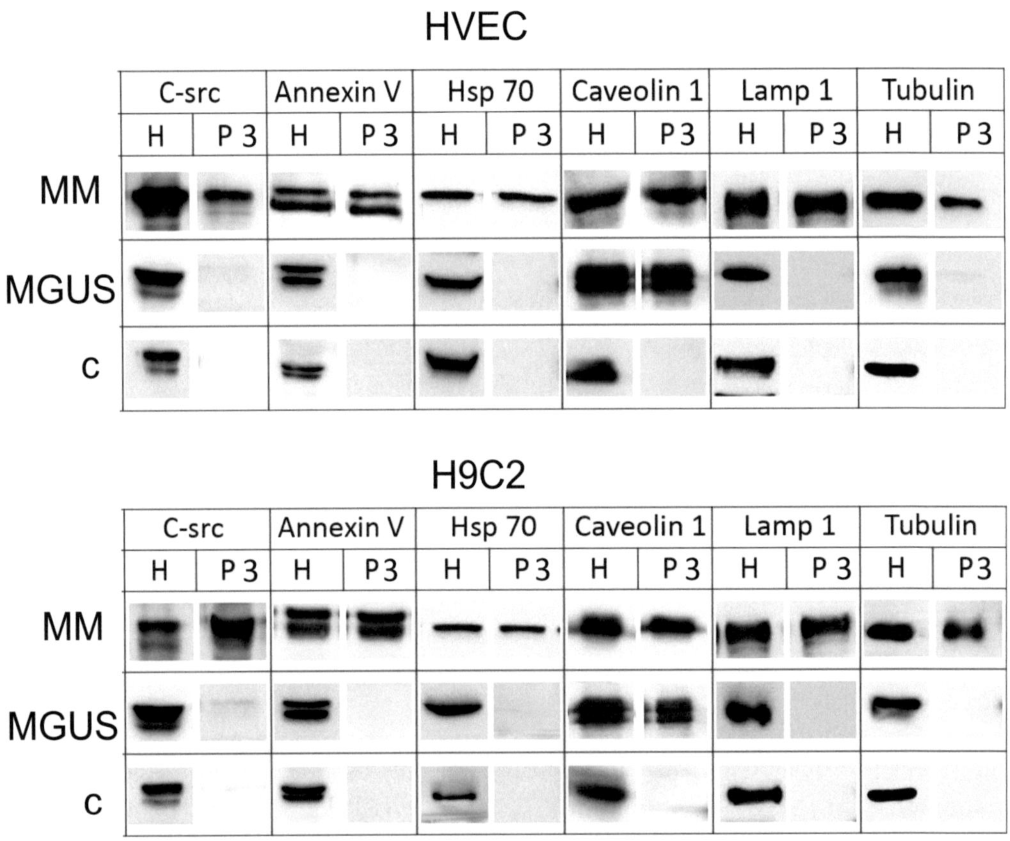

Figure 3. Biochemical characterization of cell-derived exosomes. HVEC and H9C2 cells were incubated with serum from MM, MGUS and healthy donor (c) patients for 4 h at 37°C. The serum was diluted to a final FLC concentration of 20 μg/mL for all samples. Cells were then washed with PBS 1× and treated with trypsin as described in Di Noto et al. and left in fresh medium for 16 h. Medium was harvested, centrifuged at 800 × g for 30 min, 16,000 × g for 45 min and finally, ultracentrifuged at 100,000 × g for 2 h (P3). WB analysis of cell extracts (homogenate, H) and pellets (P3) with different exosome markers (C-src, Annexin V, Hsp 70, Caveolin 1, and Lamp 1). Adapted from Di Noto et al. [10].

evidence of biochemical diversity between exosomes from cells incubated with MM and MGUS serum.

3. EVs detection in MM and MGUS patients' serum

3.1. FLC content of serum-derived EVs

One of the main disadvantages of experiments using immortalized cell lines is that it can be challenging to extrapolate from the results of *in vitro* work back to the biology of the intact organism [20].

For this reason, it was important to confirm the results obtained after studying the FLC processing in human cell lines and verify the presence of the EVs also *in vivo*, analyzing directly patients' serum. After the three step centrifugation protocol on serum, EVs were found in samples from MM and MGUS patients, and MM vesicles show a higher amount of FLC in the P3 fraction than MGUS and healthy patients, estimated around 2% of all the FLC present in serum [10]. These data are consistent with a previous study on urinary exosomes from AL amyloidosis, MM, and MGUS patients [21]. The presence of small amount of FLC in P3 of MGUS serum can be explained with the high variability of EVs production *in vivo* respect of the more restricted type of EVs deriving from a cell culture. Nevertheless, MGUS EVs present different characteristics with respect to MM EVs as explained further in the chapter.

3.2. Serum EVs biochemical characterization

Similar to exosomes from cells, EV preparations from serum must be validated by WB analysis for exosomal markers: P3 from the serum of MM and MGUS patients were blotted for Hsp70, Annexin V, and Tubulin giving positive signals. It is also to note that in the serum, the MGUS exosomes do not contain c-src, confirming that this protein is a marker of malignancy in exosomes from MM patients (**Figure 4A**) [10, 22].

3.2.1. Discontinuous sucrose gradient

Exosomes can be distinct from other type of vesicles for their density, ranging from 1.077 to 1.19 g/mL [6, 16]. Exosomes from MM serum loaded on a discontinuous sucrose gradient from 15 to 60% can be detected in four fractions (from 6 to 9) with density from 1.084 to 1.18 g/mL, according to the markers Hsp70, Annexin V, CD63, TSG101, and CD81 (**Figure 4B**) [6, 10, 22, 23]. FLC and c-src are detected in the same fractions, confirming their association with MM exosomes [10].

In our lab experience and according to guidelines [16], it is best to perform this separation with samples containing high amount of exosomes, for example serum with respect to cellular medium. Usually, exosomes spread in 4–5 gradient fractions and this dilution can decrease

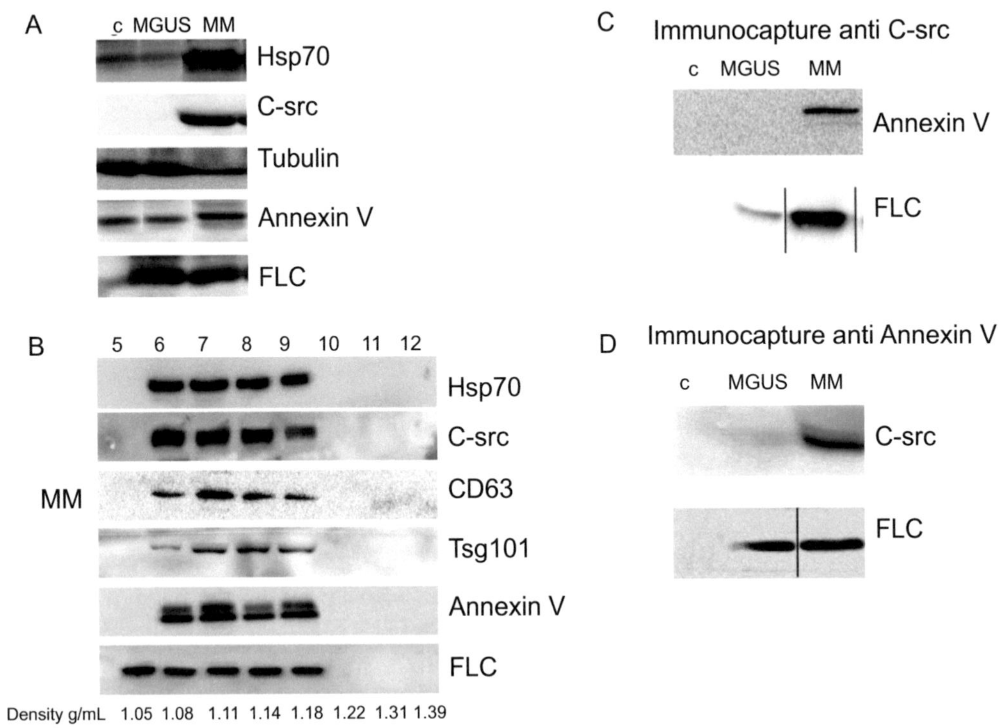

Figure 4. Serum exosome biochemical characterization. (A) P3 obtained from healthy donors (c), MGUS and MM patients were analyzed by WB with different exosome markers. (B) P3 from MM patient was loaded on top of a 15–60% discontinuous sucrose gradient. Twelve fractions of equal volume were collected and analyzed by WB using different exosomal markers and anti-FLC antibodies. Exosomal markers and FLC signals are visible in the same fractions. (C and D) P3 from healthy donors (c), MGUS and MM serum were loaded in a discontinuous sucrose gradient. Fractions from 6 to 9 were collected and incubated with magnetic beads coupled with anti c-src (C) or Annexin V (D) antibodies. Only exosomes deriving from MM serum are both c-src and Annexin V positive. Adapted from Di Noto et al. [10, 22].

the exosomes protein concentration under the limit of detection with available substrate, usually femtomolar, used for the chemiluminescent reaction in WB.

3.2.2. C-src and annexin V MM immunocapture

The immunocapture assay performed with magnetic beads coupled with antibodies anti-c-src (**Figure 4C**) confirmed the ability to precipitate only exosomes (Annexin V positive) from MM serum-containing FLC. On the other hand, anti-Annexin V beads captured MGUS and MM exosomes, but only MM exosomes were positive for c-src signal.

3.2.3. Exosome lipid composition

The lipid composition of the two exosomal populations was analyzed by a thin-layer chromatography showing that both MM and MGUS exosomes are composed by phosphatidylcholine and sphingomyelin, two well-known types of lipids that compose exosome membranes [15]. It is to note that to reveal the P3 MGUS lipids content, we loaded twice the protein concentration than MM P3 (see also Section 3.4).

3.2.4. Flow cytometry characterization

MM and MGUS exosomes were incubated with FACS magnetic beads coupled to CD63 antibody and stained with a commercial membrane labeler (PKH26). Fluorescent signal was analyzed by flow cytometry revealing the presence of exosomes with the same profile of CD63 expression level [22].

3.3. Serum exosomes morphological analysis

According to the guidelines, in addition to the biochemical characterization described above, to claim the presence of EVs, in particular exosomes, in a preparation, a "single vesicles characterization" is recommended to provide indication of the heterogeneity of the sample [16, 18].

MM and MGUS exosomes preparation both from P3 and gradient fractions were analyzed by atomic force microscopy (AFM), scanning electron microscopy (SEM), and scanning helium ion microscopy (HIM). AFM allows the analysis of vesicles that tend to remain in their original 3D shape. SEM and HIM have a better resolution, but the samples are manipulated. They need to be fixed and dehydrated and these steps can create aggregates and artifacts. In our case, however, all of these techniques allowed to visualize vesicles ranging from 50 to 300 nm according to the heterogeneity of the sample: P3 contains exosomes and bigger vesicles, while gradient fractions are more monodispersed with a size range between 50 and 150 nm (**Figure 5**).

3.4. MM and MGUS exosome quantification

Exosome quantification in a sample is one of the most discussed issues among experts in the field. How is it possible to quantify accurately something with the heterogeneous composition (lipids, protein, and nucleic acids) among a mixture of similar elements (protein aggregated from serum, circulating RNA, and vesicles with similar size, but different origin)?

Bradford assay was used to determine the amount of the total exosomes protein in the samples, and with this method, P3 from MM serum had almost double protein concentration than P3 from MGUS and healthy patients.

Further on, it has been discovered that exosome preparation protein content can be influenced by many elements, i.e. fetal bovine serum in culture medium, single, and aggregated proteins. One of the best solutions is to purify the sample as much as possible from contaminants before every type of measurements, i.e. with a sucrose gradient. Even though what is Bradford assay measuring: protein outside or inside exosomes, or both?

Thus, we decide to measure the activity of an enzyme known to be enriched within exosomes, acetylcholinesterase [24], in a P3 preparation from healthy, MGUS, and MM serum. This assay confirmed that MM P3 preparation contains more exosomes than MGUS and controls, but how much is it specific?

Our lab contributed to solve this set of problems with a nanotechnological approach. We developed a cost-effective and fast colorimetric assay for probing protein contaminants and determining the concentration of EV preparations [25].

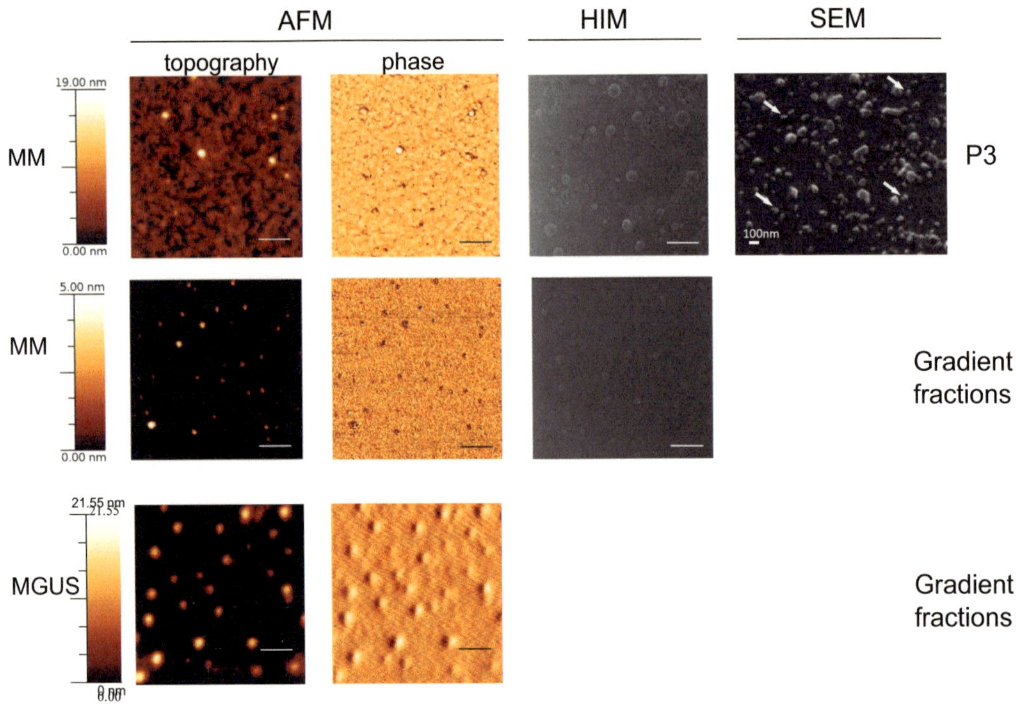

Figure 5. Serum exosome morphological analysis. P3 from MM serum were analyzed by AFM, HIM, and SEM in order to visualize vesicle populations. MM and MGUS sucrose gradient fractions from 6 to 9 were examined by AFM (topography and phase mode) and HIM (only MM sample). MM scale bars are 300 nm for AFM pictures, 500 nm for HIM pictures, and 100 nm for SEM picture. MGUS scale bars are 700 nm for AFM pictures. Adapted from Paolini et al. [6] and Di Noto et al. [10].

The assay exploits colloidal gold nanoplasmonics and the fact that nanoparticle (NP) aggregation at lipid membranes is modulated by the presence of a protein corona around the NPs. When a pure exosome preparation is incubated with a gold NP solution, the NPs cluster at the exosome membrane. Clustering is associated with NP LSPR red-shift, which is proportional to the exosome molar concentration and using a calibration line made of phosphatidylcholine liposome, can therefore be exploited for titrating the solution. If the preparation is not pure from single or aggregated proteins, NPs tend to interact with these elements and do not aggregate on exosome surface. Thus, to obtain a precise exosome quantification, as described, sample must be as pure as possible.

This assay, moreover, can determine the sample purity from protein contaminants with a limit of detection of 0.005 μg/μL.

Using this assay, we probed MM and MGUS exosomes collected from the sucrose gradient fractions from 6 to 9, and we could state that exosome preparations were pure from protein contaminants. In this way, our assay could titrate the exosome concentration in each sample and results showed a four-fold increase of exosomes in MM preparation in comparison with MGUS and healthy control (**Figure 6**) [23]. These data confirmed the previous analyses of exosomes from serum and it corresponds to the production of exosomes in the cells after MM and MGUS serum exposure.

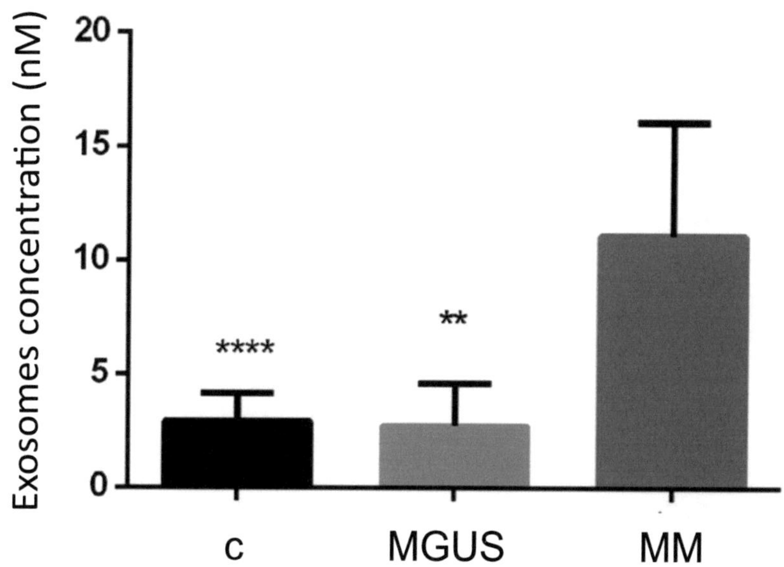

Figure 6. MM and MGUS exosome serum quantification. Exosomes were titrated using the colorimetric nanoplasmonic assay as described in Maiolo et al. [25]. Each column represents the mean value of exosomes isolated from serum of different patients (10 healthy donors (c), 5 MGUS and 10 MM) +/− Standard deviation. Student's t-test p value (p): **** p < 0,0001, *** p < 0.01. Adapted from Di Noto et al. [23].

4. MM and MGUS exosome biological effects

Exosome role in MM is started to be unveiled in the past few years. MM-derived EVs have been demonstrated to have a biological effect on other cell types, such as to induce phenotypical changes in osteoclasts, influence bone marrow microenvironment, and promote the production of proangiogenic factors, like IL-6 and VEFG, in endothelial cells [26].

Interestingly, MM and MGUS serum-derived exosomes showed different biological effects on endothelial and myocardial cell lines: MM exosomes have a higher internalization rate than MGUS and treatment with MM exosomes was able to induce a significantly higher proliferation rate compared with MGUS in both cell lines.

This effect is dependent on active exosomes endocytosis in cells, mediated by the presence of specific pathogenic FLC on the surface of MM exosome as demonstrated with immunofluorescence and cytofluorometry analyses (**Figure 7A and B**). In fact, MM exosomes incubated with antibodies anti-FLC, which mask the interaction with cells, decrease their internalization rate and the induced cell proliferation in both cell lines (**Figure 7C**). Furthermore, MM exosomes docking and processing by cells is influenced by the presence of heparan sulfate proteoglycans (HSPGs) on the cell surface. Incubating MM exosome with heparin, a structural analog of HSPGs, saccharide chains, decreased MM exosome uptake in HVEC cells. MM exosome/heparin interaction is being confirmed in dose-response experiments at surface plasmon resonance (SPR) spectroscopy. These data revealed a probably cooperative binding mechanism of FLC and HSPGs even if exosomes, which are characterized by different FLC decorations, have distinct binding affinities for cell-associated HSPGs and this is reflected in different cellular uptake [22, 23].

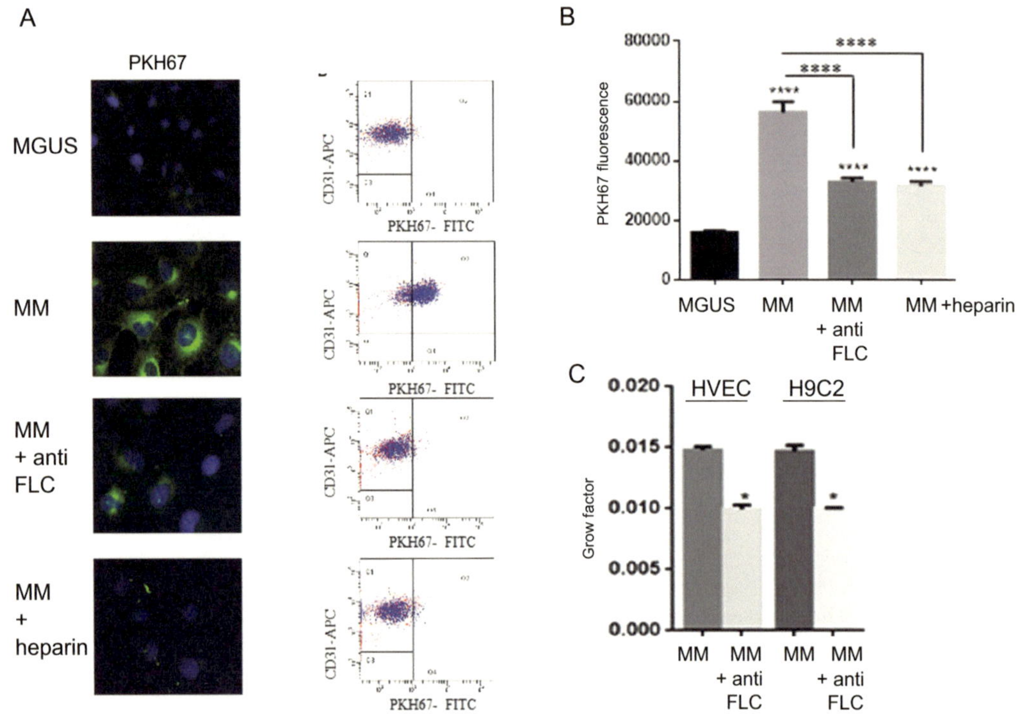

Figure 7. MM exosome biological effect is FLC and HSPG mediated. (A) Fluorescent microscopy and flow cytometry analyses of HVEC cells incubated with MGUS or MM PKH67-labeled exosomes. To demonstrate the FLC and HSPGs involvement in MM exosome uptake, MM vesicles were incubated with anti-FLC antibody (MM+ anti FLC) or heparin before cells incubation. Scale bars 5 μm. (B) PKH67 fluorescence intensity measurement of internalized exosomes from MGUS and MM serum. MM exosomes uptake in HVEC cells decrease after anti-FLC antibody (MM+ anti FLC) or heparin treatments. (C) Proliferation induction by MM exosomes is decreased after incubation with anti-FLC antibody both in HVEC and H9C2 cell lines. Adapted from Di Noto et al. [22].

It has been demonstrated that MM EVs are related to proinflammatory environment in cells. Immunofluorescence and biochemical separation techniques demonstrated that cells treated with exosomes from MM serum show a c-src intracellular redistribution at the plasma membrane with respect to MGUS exosome treatment. These data are consistent with cellular *ex novo* secretion of c-src positive exosomes after MM serum exposure and this phenomenon is reduced after cellular uptake inhibition, incubating MM exosomes with anti-FLC antibodies and heparin.

Similarly, the activation and nuclear translocation of the transcription factor Nf-kB, involved in the cellular responses after stress, infection, and inflammatory stimuli, is not visible in the cell treated with MGUS exosomes. MM exosome's induced effect is decreased after treatment with anti-FLC antibody and heparin (**Figure 8**).

It is to note that the Nf-kB translocation is dependent on the preparation purity: the biological activity of exosome preparations from MM patient serum is influenced by residual contaminants, which may escape the purification procedure. These contaminants probably can interfere with the exosomes-cell membrane interaction or inhibit the Nf-kB translocation. They can be

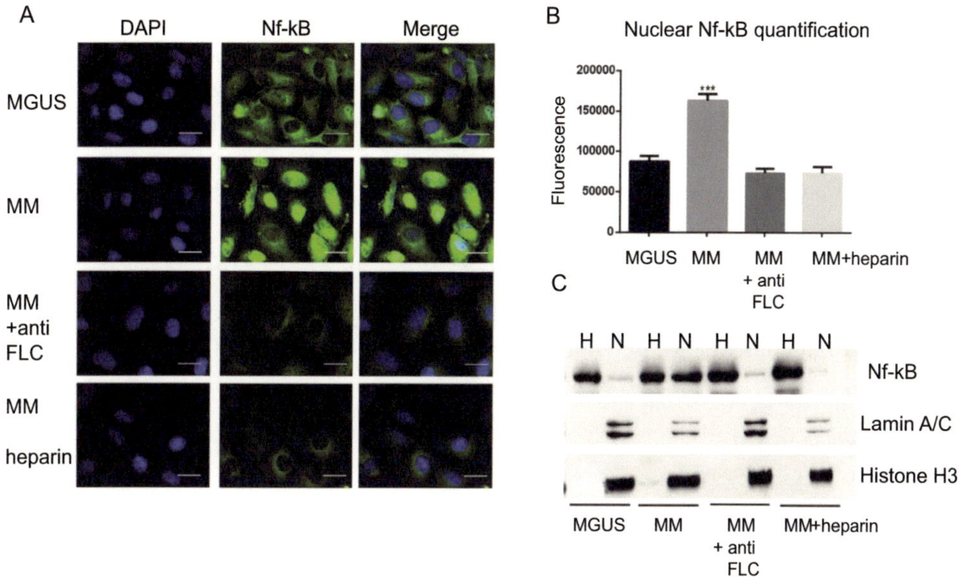

Figure 8. Nf-kB nuclear translocation is MM exosomes induced. (A) HVEC immunofluorescence imaging of Nf-kB nuclear translocation after incubation with MGUS, MM exosomes, or MM exosomes incubated with anti-FLC antibody (MM + anti FLC) or heparin (MM + heparin). Cell were fixed and incubated with DAPI for nuclear staining and anti-Nf-kB antibody as described in Di Noto et al. [22]. Scale bars 5 μm. (B) Quantification of nuclear Nf-kB fluorescence intensity in HVEC cells after MGUS, MM exosomes, MM exosomes incubated with anti-FLC antibody (MM + anti FLC) or with heparin (MM + heparin) treatment. (C) WB analysis of cell extracts (H) and nuclear compartment (N) was performed with anti Nf-kB antibody and nuclear markers (Lamin A/C, Histone H3) after different incubations. Adapted from Di Noto et al. [22].

separated from exosomes after a discontinuous gradient, but they cannot be detected with conventional techniques (i.e. WB) and need a combination of proper bioanalytical methods and nanoscale characterization [6].

5. Conclusion

In this chapter, we have shown that MM and MGUS patients can be distinguished at the nanoscale level. Although their FLC serum content may be similar, FLC biochemical characteristics are very different: they are internalized and processed in cells in distinct ways and only pathogenic FLCs are rerouted in the extracellular compartment in c-src positive exosomes. It is important to note that exosome presenting MM FLC activates a proinflammatory process: the presence of circulating c-src positive exosomes has been demonstrated only in serum of MM patients, electing this kinase as a new marker of malignancy for the differential diagnosis between MGUS and MM. Similarly only MM exosomes have the ability to induce Nf-kB translocation in cells. These parameters could be implemented with the exosome concentration in serum, binding affinity with heparin and ability to induce proliferation in HVEC and H9C2 cell lines to create an innovative multiparameter panels to monitor MGUS to MM switching. We are aware that these data need to be confirmed in a larger cohort of patients and we still do not know how precocious these phenomena are with respect to the MGUS to MM switch using of the actual diagnostic criteria. Recently, new biomarkers are emerging to help clinicians to distinguish MM from the premalignant phase. According to recent guidelines, extreme bone marrow clonal plasmacytosis (>60%), marked elevation of serum FLC ratio of 100 or higher (provided involved free light-chain level ≥100 mg/L) and/or presence of more than one focal lesion on whole-body magnetic resonance imaging (MRI) can defined as MM even in the absence of CRAB features [2, 3].

In the future, monitoring MGUS and MM exosome parameters could support, as a liquid biopsy, the classical classification methods and help in early diagnosis to prevent the development of end-organ damage for patients who are at the highest risk [2, 3].

Acknowledgements

We thank all the colleagues that contribute to this work: Annalisa Radeghieri, Sara Busatto, Daniele Maiolo, Debora Berti, Elisa Polini, Elisabetta Lottini, Marco Chiarini, Elena Laura Mazzoldi, Viviana Giustini, Alessandra Dossi, Antonella Bugatti, Alesssandro Montanelli, Marco Rusnati, Andrea Caneschi, and Luigi Caimi. This work was supported by the University of Brescia Research through the found "ex 60%" and by MIUR (Ministero Italiano dell'Università e della Ricerca). Fondazione Cariplo and Regione Lombardia supported the publication through the found "New Opportunities and ways towards ERC", grant 2014–2256. The authors declare no conflict of interests.

Author details

Lucia Paolini*, Giuseppe Di Noto, Andrea Zendrini, Paolo Bergese and Doris Ricotta

*Address all correspondence to: paolinilu@gmail.com

Department of Molecular and Translational Medicine, University of Brescia, Brescia, Italy

References

[1] Kyle RA, Rajkumar SV. Epidemiology of the plasma-cell disorders. Best Practice & Research Clinical Haematology. 2007;**20**(4):637-664

[2] Rajkumar SV, Dimopoulos MA, Palumbo A, Blade J, Merlini G, Mateos MV, Kumar S, Hillengass J, Kastritis E, Richardson P, Landgren O, Paiva B, Dispenzieri A, Weiss B, LeLeu X, Zweegman S, Lonial S, Rosinol L, Zamagni E, Jagannath S, Sezer O, Kristinsson SY, Caers J, Usmani SZ, Lahuerta JJ, Johnsen HE, Beksac M, Cavo M, Goldschmidt H,

Terpos E, Kyle RA, Anderson KC, Durie BG, Miguel JF. International Myeloma Working Group updated criteria for the diagnosis of multiple myeloma. Lancet Oncology. 2014;**15**(12):e538–e548. DOI: 10.1016/S1470-2045(14)70442-5

[3] Rajkumar SV. Updated diagnostic criteria and staging system for multiple myeloma. American Society of Clinical Oncology Educational Book. 2016;**35**:e418-e423. DOI: 10.14694/EDBK_159009

[4] Pantel K, Dive C. Liquid Biopsy in the Clinic. 2016 [Internet]. Available from http://www.nature.com/nrclinonc/posters/liquidbiopsies/nrclinonc_liquidbiopsies_poster_web.pdf [Accessed: February 23, 2017]

[5] Sánchez-Vela P, Garcia NA, Campos-Segura M, Forteza-Vila J. Liquid biopsy and tumor-derived exosomes in clinical practice. Revista Española de Patología. 2016;**49**:106-111. DOI: 10.1016/j.patol.2015.11.004

[6] Paolini L, Zendrini A, Di Noto G, Busatto S, Lottini E, Radeghieri A, Dossi A, Caneschi A, Ricotta D, Bergese P. Residual matrix from different separation techniques impacts exosome biological activity. Scientific Reports. 2016;**6**:23550. DOI: 10.1038/srep23550

[7] Manier S, Liu CJ, Avet-Loiseau H, Park J, Shi J, Campigotto F, Salem KZ, Huynh D, Glavey SV, Rivotto B, Sacco A, Roccaro AM, Bouyssou J, Minvielle S, Moreau P, Facon T, Leleu X, Weller E, Trippa L, Ghobrial IM. Prognostic role of circulating exosomal miRNAs in multiple myeloma. Blood. 2017;**129**:2429-2436. DOI: 10.1182/blood-2016-09-742296

[8] Dispenzieri A, Kyle R, Merlini G, Miguel JS, Ludwig H, Hajek R, Palumbo A, Jagannath S, Blade J, Lonial S, Dimopoulos M, Comenzo R, Einsele H, Barlogie B, Anderson K, Gertz M, Harousseau JL, Attal M, Tosi P, Sonneveld P, Boccadoro M, Morgan G, Richardson P, Sezer O, Mateos MV, Cavo M, Joshua D, Turesson I, Chen W, Shimizu K, Powles R, Rajkumar SV, Durie BG, International Myeloma Working Group. International Myeloma Working Group guidelines for serum-free light chain analysis in multiple myeloma and related disorders. Leukemia. 2009;**23**(2):215-224. DOI: 10.1038/leu.2008.307

[9] Di Noto G, Cimpoies E, Dossi A, Paolini L, Radeghieri A, Caimi L, Ricotta D. Polyclonal versus monoclonal immunoglobulin-free light chains quantification. Annals of Clinical Biochemistry: International Journal of Laboratory Medicine. 2015;**52**:327-336. DOI: 10.1177/0004563214553808

[10] Di Noto G, Paolini L, Zendrini A, Radeghieri A, Caimi L, Ricotta D. C-src enriched serum microvesicles are generated in malignant plasma cell dyscrasia. PLoS One. 2013;**8**(8):e70811. DOI: 10.1371/journal.pone.0070811

[11] van de Donk NW, Palumbo A, Johnsen HE, Engelhardt M, Gay F, Gregersen H, Hajek R, Kleber M, Ludwig H, Morgan G, Musto P, Plesner T, Sezer O, Terpos E, Waage A, Zweegman S, Einsele H, Sonneveld P, Lokhorst HM, European Myeloma Network. The clinical relevance and management of monoclonal gammopathy of undetermined significance and related disorders: Recommendations from the European Myeloma Network. Haematologica. 2014;**99**(6):984-996. DOI: 10.3324/haematol.2013.100552

[12] Lavatelli F, Brambilla F, Valentini V, Rognoni P, Casarini S, Di Silvestre D, Perfetti V, Palladini G, Sarais G, Mauri P, Merlini G. A novel approach for the purification and proteomic analysis of pathogenic immunoglobulin free light chains from serum. Biochimica et Biophysica Acta (BBA)—Proteins and Proteomics. 2011;**1814**(3):409-419. DOI: 10.1016/j.bbapap.2010.12.012

[13] Ricotta D, Di Noto G, Dossi A, Paolini L, Radeghieri A, Amoroso B, Caimi L. Internalization pathway of amiloydogenic Serum Free Light Chains. In: Poster Communication at 6th International Symposium on Clinical Applications of Serum Free Light Chain Analysis (plus Hevylite); 23rd and 24th September 2010. Bath, UK

[14] Ren R, Hong Z, Gong H, Laporte K, Skinner M, Seldin DC, Costello CE, Connors LH, Trinkaus-Randall V. Role of glycosaminoglycan sulfation in the formation of immunoglobulin light chain amyloid oligomers and fibrils. Journal of Biological Chemistry. 2010;**285**(48):37672-37682. DOI: 10.1074/jbc.M110.149575

[15] Maas SL, Breakefield XO, Weaver AM. Extracellular vesicles: Unique intercellular delivery vehicles. Trends in Cell Biology. 2017;**27**(3):172-188. DOI: 10.1016/j.tcb.2016.11.003

[16] Théry C, Amigorena S, Raposo G, Clayton A. Isolation and characterization of exosomes from cell culture supernatants and biological fluids. Current Protocols in Cell Biology. 2006. Chapter 3:Unit 3.22. DOI: 10.1002/0471143030.cb0322s30

[17] Soung YH, Ford S, Zhang V, Chung J. Exosomes in cancer diagnostics. Cancers. 2017;**9**(1): 8-19. DOI: 10.3390/cancers9010008

[18] Lötvall J, Hill AF, Hochberg F, Buzás EI, Di Vizio D, Gardiner C, Gho YS, Kurochkin IV, Mathivanan S, Quesenberry P, Sahoo S, Tahara H, Wauben MH, Witwer KW, Théry C. Minimal experimental requirements for definition of extracellular vesicles and their functions: A position statement from the International Society for Extracellular Vesicles. The Journal of Extracellular Vesicles. 2014;**3**:26913. DOI: 10.3402/jev.v3.26913

[19] Heusschen R, Muller J, Binsfeld M, Marty C, Plougonven E, Dubois S, Mahli N, Moermans K, Carmeliet G, Léonard A, Baron F, Beguin Y, Menu E, Cohen-Solal M, Caers J. SRC kinase inhibition with saracatinib limits the development of osteolytic bone disease in multiple myeloma. Oncotarget. 2016;**7**(21):30712-30729. DOI: 10.18632/oncotarget.8750

[20] Rothman SS. Lessons from the Living Cell: The Culture of Science and the Limits of Reductionism. New York: McGraw-Hill; 2002. ISBN 0-07-137820-0

[21] Ramirez-Alvarado M, Ward CJ, Huang BQ, Gong X, Hogan MC, Madden BJ, Charlesworth MC, Leung N. Differences in immunoglobulin light chain species found in urinary exosomes in light chain amyloidosis (Al). PLoS One. 2012;**7**(6):e38061. DOI: 10.1371/journal.pone.0038061

[22] Di Noto G, Chiarini M, Paolini L, Mazzoldi EL, Giustini V, Radeghieri A, Caimi L, Ricotta D. Immunoglobulin free light chains and GAGs mediate multiple myeloma extracellular vesicles uptake and secondary NfκB nuclear translocation. Frontiers in Immunology. 2014;**5**:517. DOI: 10.3389/fimmu.2014.00517

[23] Di Noto G, Bugatti A, Zendrini A, Mazzoldi EL, Montanelli A, Caimi L, Rusnati M, Ricotta D, Bergese P. Merging colloidal nanoplasmonics and surface plasmon resonance spectroscopy for enhanced profiling of multiple myeloma-derived exosomes. Biosensors and Bioelectronics. 2016;**77**:518-524. DOI: 10.1016/j.bios.2015.09.061

[24] Savina A, Vidal M, Colombo MI. The exosome pathway in K562 cells is regulated by Rab11. The Journal of Cell Science. 2002;**115**:2505-2515

[25] Maiolo D, Paolini L, Di Noto G, Zendrini A, Berti D, Bergese P, Ricotta D. Colorimetric nanoplasmonic assay to determine purity and titrate extracellular vesicles. Analytical Chemistry. 2015;**87**(8):4168-4176. DOI: 10.1021/ac504861d

[26] Canella A, Harshman SW, Radomska HS, Freitas MA, Pichiorri F. The potential diagnostic power of extracellular vesicle analysis for multiple myeloma. Expert Review of Molecular Diagnostics. 2016;**16**(3):277-84. DOI: 10.1586/14737159.2016.1132627

Chapter 3

Animal Models in Exosomes Research: What the Future Holds

Bárbara Adem and Sónia A. Melo

Additional information is available at the end of the chapter

http://dx.doi.org/10.5772/intechopen.69449

Abstract

Exosomes have been implicated in a wide range of pathological and nonpathological processes. Research on tumor-derived exosomes uncovered their role on major processes associated with disease progression. Uncontrolled cellular proliferation resulting in tumor growth, metastatic dissemination and modulation of the immune response, are only a few of the central pathological processes in which tumor-derived exosomes have been implicated. These *in vivo* studies rely on the administration of purified labeled exosomes from cell culture supernatants into circulation of animals or injections of genetically engineered cells that produce labeled exosomes. However, it is not clear that current available techniques actually translate the *in vivo* implications of exosomes in several biological processes. The variations seen when using different exosomes cell sources, the total amount of exosomes injected in mice and their route of administration as well as the fact that most studies are performed in immunodeficient animals, shows the difficulty to achieve conclusions which are biologically significant. Genetically engineered mouse models (GEMM) could be a promising approach to address the current technical limitations allowing tracing tumor-derived exosomes in a living organism. These models could enhance greatly our knowledge about exosomes in different fields of research, namely cancer.

Keywords: exosomes, biodistribution, labeling, *in vivo* imaging, tumor progression

1. Introduction

During the last decades, extensive research on exosomes has contributed to the increasing knowledge on their composition, biogenesis and biological function [1]. Exosomes intrinsic ability of horizontal cargo transfer, and their high stability in circulation, allows them to interact with neighbor and distant cells and phenotypically reprogram them, being important mediators of cell-to-cell communication [2]. Numerous *in vitro* studies clearly demonstrate exosomes ability to modulate recipient cells through the transfer of their cargo, which includes proteins, DNA and RNA [3–7]. Much effort has been made to evaluate exosomes biological significance *in vivo* through the study of how they flow inside a multicellular organism, their fate upon exocytosis and in which cells they enter and what changes they elicit. Various

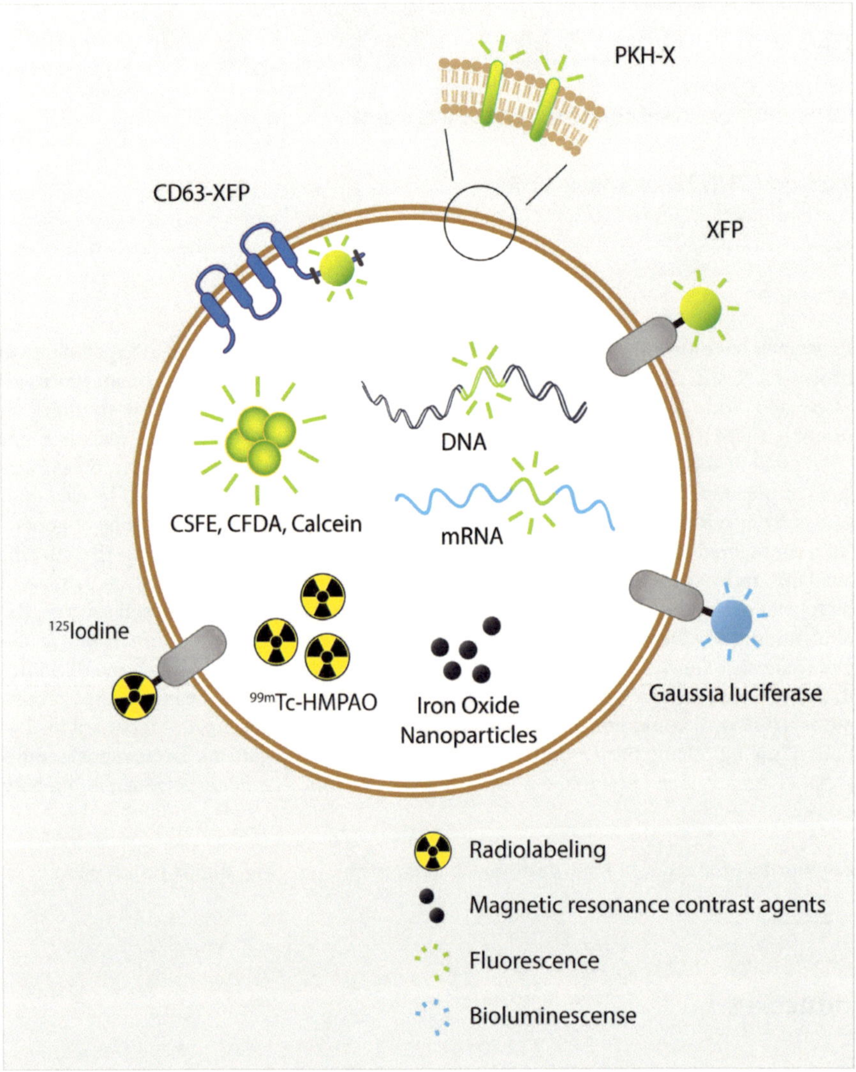

Figure 1. Exosomes biodistribution studies are based on two main approaches: administration of labeled exosomes into circulation of animals, previously extracted from cell culture supernatants, or injections of genetically engineered cells that produce labeled exosomes. Most of the studies performed thus far make use of exogenously produced exosomes isolated from cell culture medium, following injection by different routes of administration, including intraperitoneal (i.p.), intravenous (i.v.), subcutaneous (s.c.), retro-orbital, intranasal and *via* footpad to further track exosomes fate *in vivo*. The other approach consists of injecting subcutaneously or orthotopically cells that had been genetically engineered in order to produce labeled exosomes. This last method allows the track of both cells and corresponding exosomes within the tumor microenvironment or at distant sites.

studies have tried several imaging techniques to track exosomes fate *in vivo* in order to dissect communication routes and their biological implications. Studies conducted so far have described a central role for exosomes in the establishment of the pre-metastatic niche, as well as their close interaction with the immune system [8–12]. Despite latest findings, understanding their spatio-temporal distribution and physiological functions *in vivo* remains a major challenge in the field. Actually, the biological functions of exosomes *in vivo*, including tissue distribution, blood levels and clearance dynamics remain largely unexplored.

Exosomes biodistribution research is based on two main approaches: administration of purified labeled exosomes from cell culture supernatants into circulation of animals or injections of genetically engineered cells that produce labeled exosomes (**Figure 1**). According to the literature, most studies performed so far used exogenously produced exosomes isolated from cell culture medium, following treatment using different routes of administration, including intraperitoneal (i.p.), intravenous (i.v.), subcutaneous (s.c.), retro-orbital, intranasal and *via* footpad to further track exosomes fate *in vivo* [10, 13–15]. To successfully follow exosomes

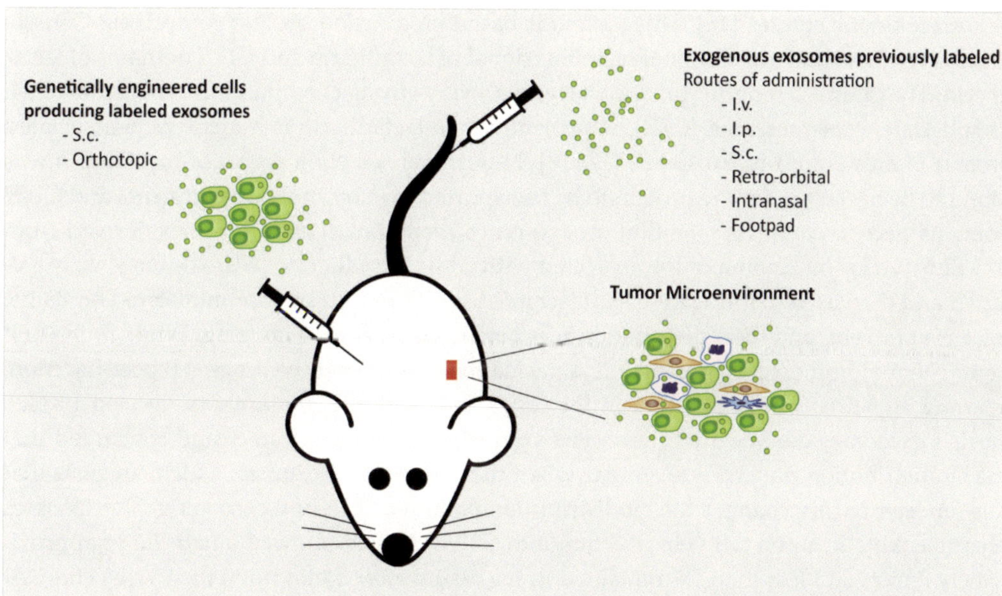

Figure 2. Different methods available to label exosomes. Fluorescent labeling of exosomes is the most widely used method to trace their fate *in vivo*. Membrane-intercalating fluorescent dyes such as PKH or PKH26 are very common. Fluorescent probes labeling DNA, mRNA and proteins contained in exosomes are also an option. Additionally, membrane permeable fluorescent dyes as carboxyfluorescein succinimidyl ester (CFSE), 5(6)-carboxyfluorescein diacetate (CFDA) and calcein fluoresce as a consequence of esterification. Furthermore, exosomes labeling resulting of the genetic engineering of the cells of origin are also a common approach. Fluorescent reporters can be fused to exosomes markers like CD63. Fluorescent labeling can be detected using standard optical imaging techniques. Other labeling systems have been developed such as the bioluminescence reporters like gaussia luciferase fused to transmembrane domains of known proteins like lactadherin or platelet-derived growth factor receptor. Other options include radiolabeling of exosomes using ^{125}Iodine to label exosomal proteins located on the outer membrane or by using ^{99m}Tc-hexamethylpropyleneamineo (HMPAO) that can be visualized using single-photon emission computed tomography. Exosomes labeling with magnetic resonance contrast agents such as iron oxide nanoparticles is an innovative approach and further tracking can be achieved through magnetic resonance imaging.

fate *in vivo*, labeling methods should satisfy the following requirements: (1) specifically label exosomes rather than extracellular vesicles (EVs) in general; (2) be stable and accumulate sufficient signal to detect exosomes from background noise; (3) not interfere with exosomes natural half-life; and (4) not alter exosomes properties. Taking these into consideration, several methods have been developed to labels EVs, namely exosomes (**Figure 2**).

2. Bioluminescence reporter system

Genetically engineered bioluminescent proteins such as Gaussia luciferase, combined with transmembrane domains like lactadherin- or platelet-derived growth factor receptor (PDGFR), could reveal the spatiotemporal distribution of EVs in a quantitative manner in small animals [14, 16]. This approach overcomes the limitation of background auto-fluorescence when working with fluorescent proteins. Nevertheless, this system presents the disadvantage of attenuated signal when located in a deep organ. In 2013, Takahashi et al. designed a new reporter system based on bioluminescence that enables tissue biodistribution and pharmacokinetic studies [16]. This system is based on a fusion protein comprising Gaussia luciferase (gLuc) and a N-terminal secretion signal of lactadherin and C1C2 domains of lactadherin. The gLuc is a reporter protein that emits a very strong chemiluminescent signal when its substrate, coelenterazine (CTZ), is present, while lactadherin is a membrane-associated protein mainly found in exosomes [17, 18]. N-terminal secretion signal of lactadherin was found to be necessary for the protein to be transported to exosomal compartments and C1C2 domains necessary for its retention on exosomes membrane [18]. Exosomes derived from B16-BL6 murine melanoma cells transfected with GLuc lactadherine (GL exosomes) were collected and then used to intravenously inject mice. GL exosomes were administered on Balb/c mice *via* tail vein, and their distribution was evaluated by *in vivo* imaging. While in the first hour, chemioluminescence was mainly detected in the liver and the lungs, 4 h post-injection, a strong signal was only detected in the lungs. Interestingly, the authors injected PKH26 labeled exosomes derived from nontransfected B16-BL6 cells into mice and concluded that the biodistribution pattern was similar when they used GL exosomes, which suggests that this reporter hardly changes the biodistribution pattern of B16-BL6 exosomes. GL exosomes pharmacokinetic, upon tail vein injection into C57/BL6 mice, showed a half-life of approximately 2 min, and less than 5% remained in the serum after 5 min upon the i.v. injection. At 4 h upon injection, strong gLuc activity was detected in the lungs and spleen [16]. Further studies developed by the same group investigated the clearance mechanism of i.v. injected B16BL6 GL exosomes [19]. PKH26-labeled B16BL6 exosomes were taken up by macrophages present in the liver and spleen and by endothelial cells in the lung. To assess the role of macrophages in exosomes clearance, B16BL6 GL exosomes were i.v. injected into macrophage-depleted mice. In those animals, exosomes clearance was significantly delayed, and levels were reduced to around 1.6% comparing to the untreated mice. Collectively, these findings demonstrate that macrophages play a preponderant role in the clearance of injected exosomes from the blood circulation.

Lai et al. also developed an additional multimodal reporter for EVs imaging based on bioluminescence [14]. A recombinant protein composed of a transmembrane domain of PDGFR

http://dx.doi.org/10.5772/intechopen.69449

fused to a biotin acceptor domain that is fused to the humanized Gaussia luciferase was expressed in the membranes of EVs. In the presence of coelenterazine (CTZ), the purified vesicles exhibited a strong bioluminescent signal. When conjugated to streptavidin-Alexa 680, the EVs can be imaged *in vivo* noninvasively using several techniques: magnetic resonance imaging (MRI), single-photon emission computed tomography/positron emission tomography (SPEC/PET) and fluorescence-mediated tomography (FMT). Stable clones of HEK293T cells expressing both the recombinant protein and the humanized biotin ligase were used to collect the modified EV, and to systemically inject in nude mice, upon which their biodistribution and clearance were evaluated. EV-gLucB or Phosphate-buffered saline (PBS) was injected into athymic nude mice *via* the retro-orbital vein. Immediately before imaging, CTZ was administered revealing a great amount of gLuc signal in the spleen and liver in EV-gLucB treated mice when compared to the controls group. To further investigate the multimodals imaging capability, EV-gLucB or PBS was labeled with streptavidin-Alexa 680 conjugate and then injected *via* tail vein into athymic nude mice and imaged 30 min later with FMT. Similarly to the biodistribution seen by gLuc bioluminescence, EVs were found to accumulate mainly in the spleen and liver. To assess biodistribution of i.v. administered EV-gLucB, organs were collected at different time points post-treatment and gLuc activity was analyzed. The highest signal was detected in the spleen, followed by the liver, lungs and kidney, which is in agreement with the *in vivo* results. On the other hand, the brain, heart and muscle showed lower amounts of signal across all time points. Interestingly, EVs signal decreased by more than half from 30 to 60 min in the liver and the kidneys, while during the same period, spleen and lung levels remained constant. In another experiment, EV-treated animals were transcardially perfused with PBS before harvesting the organs at different time points. Notably, perfused kidneys showed the highest EV signal followed by liver, lung, heart, brain, muscle, and finally, the spleen showing the lowest signal amounts across all time points. These findings suggest that cells that compose the spleen, even though high amounts of EVs are present in the blood that supplies this organ, do not efficiently take up EVs. The prevalent EVs localization in the nonperfused spleen is most likely attributed to an excess of EVs dosage resulting in the saturation of liver macrophages, leading to higher levels of EVs in circulation and consequently into spleen vasculature. Other possibility renders from the fact that EVs can be taken up in the blood by macrophages or lymphocytes that travel to the spleen. Perfused liver and lungs displayed similar reduction patterns from 30 to 60 min when compared to the nonperfused scenario indicating that these organs actively take up EVs. A similar trend was found to the brain, heart and muscle demonstrating that these organs take up EVs although in small amounts. Even though the kidneys displayed the highest amounts of vesicles accumulation, authors called our attention to a possible artifact of the perfusion procedure. In this case, EVs present in the blood would be forced into the kidneys. To study EVs kinetics in biofluids, blood and urine were collected at different time points post EV injection, and luciferase activity was evaluated. The maximum signal was detected at 30 min (earliest time point), followed by a quick reduction at 60 min and then a slow decline from 90 to 360 min. In the urine, the highest signal was measured at 60 min followed by a fast decrease from 60 to 120 min and then a progressive decline from 120 to 360 min. Altogether these findings suggest that only a minor part of EV-gLucB is cleared by the renal route upon the distribution phase. At the last time point, baseline signal was detected in the blood, whereas the urine in addition to some organs still showed part of the signal. Finally, in order to study the potential delivery of EV-gLucB to tumors, athymic nude mice with a subcutaneous human xenograft tumor were injected *via* tail vein with EV-gLucB. One hour post-treatment bioluminescence imaging revealed EV-gLucB accumulation in the tumor. When comparing liver, spleen and tumors gLuc activity, tumors were found to exhibit the highest gLuc levels. Overall, this was the first time a multimodal approach to label EVs was used giving insight into vesicles biodistribution and kinetics.

3. Radiolabeling of exosomes

In 2014, Morishita et al. developed a method to quantitatively assess the biodistribution of B16BL6-derived exosomes using iodine-125 (^{125}I) labeling on a streptavidin (SAV)-biotin system [20]. B16BL6 cells were transfected with a plasmid vector encoding the fusion protein SAV-lacadherin, and the resulting exosomes were purified and incubated with (3-^{125}I-iodobenzoyl) norbiotinamide (^{125}I-IBB) to obtain ^{125}I labeled exosomes. Balb/c mice were i.v. injected with ^{125}I labeled B16BL6 exosomes or control conditions. ^{125}I labeled B16BL6 exosomes first underwent a distribution step with a half-life of 1.5 min and then entered a clearance phase with a half-life of 346 min, indicating that exogenously administered exosomes have short half-lives in circulation. Furthermore, ^{125}I labeled B16BL6 exosomes were found to distribute to the liver, spleen and lung after systemic administration. High levels of radioactivity signal were found in the liver at 1 min, reaching a peak at 30 min and following a decrease at 4 h. Spleen distribution pattern was the same as the liver though at lower levels. Liver and spleen make part of the mononuclear phagocyte system, which is rich in macrophages and potentially responsible for the clearance of exosomes. Notably, at 1 min, a considerable amount of radioactivity was detected in the lungs, which had its peak at 1 h and decreased at 4 h. This can be due to exosomes aggregation possibly through interaction with blood components. Authors concluded that radiolabeling of exosomes with iodine-125 using the SAV-biotin system is a better choice when quantitatively determining exosomes tissue biodistribution than approaches based on fluorescence or chemioluminescence.

Additional methods have been developed to radiolabel exosomes. Hwang et al. produced exosomes-mimetic nanovesicles (ENVs) from extrusion of macrophage cells and radiolabeled them with ^{99m}Tc-hexamethylpropyleneamineo (HMPAO) under physiologic conditions [21]. The conversion of ^{99m}Tc-HMPAO in the hydrophilic form that is confined inside cells is accomplished by intracellular glutathione [22]. Further monitoring of ENVs *in vivo* biodistribution was achieved by using SPECT/CT. Biodistribution results of this particular study are not relevant to the matter reviewed in this chapter since ENVs emerged as an alternative to obtain a greater yield of exosomes in a therapeutic point of view [23]. Later, Varga et al. described a new method for radioisotope labeling of EVs using the previous mentioned ^{99m}Tc-HMPAO complex. Moreover, authors demonstrated this methods applicability for the noninvasive evaluation of the tissue distribution of erythrocyte-derived EVs using SPECT/CT [24]. The ^{99m}Tc-HMPAO complex is known to bind to some amino acids including histidine, methionine and cysteine [25]. Therefore, it was expected that this complex would bind to the surface of EVs since it presents numerous membrane proteins. Interestingly, i.v. injection of ^{99m}Tc-tricarbonyl labeled erythrocyte EVs accumulated mostly in the liver and spleen.

4. Labeling exosomes with magnetic resonance contrast agents

Studies performed by Hood group in 2014 described a new electroporation method to load mouse B16-F10 melanoma-derived exosomes with super-magnetic iron oxide nanoparticles (SPION5) [26]. This study was in agreement with their previous findings demonstrating that melanoma exosomes appear to home to the subcapsular sinus in lymph nodes (LN) [10]. Since a right and left pair of popliteal (PO) and inguinal (IN) lymph nodes drains mouse feet, they serve as sentinel LN for footpad tumors. Authors found that animals treated with SPION5 loaded exosomes exhibited a growth in the cross-sectional area of ipsilateral peripheral LN when compared to pre-treatment with free SPION5, probably due to the activation of inflammatory signaling pathways. Moreover, at the 48-h time point, the accumulation of SPION5 in the ipsilateral node was higher for SPION5 loaded exosomes compared to free SPION5. Furthermore, nodes treated with SPION5 loaded exosomes did not display significant differences in the MRI signal when comparing pre-injection and 1-h post-injection conditions. Altogether, these findings demonstrate that a greater amount of SPION5 accumulates in the ipsilateral LN when distributed by exosomes, and that exosomes need more time to deliver SPION5 to the LN than the trafficking time of free SPION5. These observations suggest that exosomes home and stay trapped in sentinel LN. Contrarily, free SPION5 and liposomes follow an unspecific diffusion throughout the LN system. The predominant subcapsular distribution of exosomes carrying SPION5 was further validated by histological analysis with fluorescence microscopy and transmission electron microscopy (TEM).

In 2016, Busato et al. established a new protocol to label exosomes with ultrasmall super-magnetic iron oxide nanoparticles (USPIO) [27]. USPIO range in size from 5 to 7 nm and are stable and biocompatible [28]. The authors described a new methodology in which adipose stem cells (ASCs) were directly labeled with USPIO rather than exosomes. ASCs are known to incorporate USPIO as part of the endocytic pathway [29]. Furthermore, other studies reported nanoparticles accumulation inside multivesicular bodies, being consequently incorporated into exosomes [30]. This protocol allows the preservation of the integrity of exosomes membrane, since no electroporation is required. The resulting exosomes were isolated, purified and injected in mice intramuscularly. Histological examination of gastrocnemius confirmed the presence of iron and *in vivo* imaging with MRI revealed to be a successful tool to image exosomes *in vivo* in a noninvasive manner.

5. Fluorescent labeling of exosomes

When administering exogenous preparations of exosomes to assess their biodistribution *in vivo*, they need to be first labeled, which can be achieved by using fluorescence techniques.

5.1. Nucleic acids labeling

The use of fluorescent dyes or fluorescent reporters has been one of the gold standard approaches to label exosomes. In addition to proteins, exosomes have been shown to carry RNA and DNA [31]. Therefore, exosomes can be fluorescently labeled using selective dyes for those nucleic acids. The SYTO 13 dye is cell permeable and has a high fluorescent yield when bound to DNA or RNA [32]. Other DNA binding dyes include H33342 and Thiazole Orange [33]. Alvarez-Erviti et al. research is one good example of this approach since they detect fluorescent signals in the central nervous system after i.v. injection of exosomes derived from dendritic cells (DC) genetically engineered to express RGV peptide on the membrane and loaded with siRNA fluorescently labeled with Cy-3 dye [34].

5.2. Membrane-intercalating fluorescent dyes

Exosomes labeling can also be achieved by using fluorescent lipid membrane dyes, including the commonly used PKH (PKH67, PKH26), which label cell membranes through the insertion of their aliphatic chains into the lipid bilayer [8, 11, 12]. Rhodamine B also known as R18, DiI, DiO and DiD, in addition to PKH, are other examples of lipophilic fluorescent membrane dyes [35–37]. The carbocyanine dyes, DiI (yellow/red fluorescent) and DiO (green fluorescent), are weakly fluorescent in aqueous solutions but become highly fluorescent and reasonably photo-stable when incorporated into cell membranes particularly, DiR (carbocyanine DiOC18(7)) [33]. A limitation for *in vivo* tracking studies is the fact that fluorescent markers should have an emission peak different from the fluorescence emission of biological tissues, in order to overcome the auto-fluorescence background. Notably, near-infrared (NIR) dyes are optimal for *in vivo* applications since they present a high signal/noise ratio, a negligible auto-fluorescence in the range of 700–900 nm (biological tissues emission), and strong tissue penetration of the NIR light [38]. However, lipophilic dyes labeling presents several limitations. Extensive washing steps are necessary to reduce unspecific signal, which can cause significant exosomes loss. Moreover, it promotes aggregates or micelles and may give rise to *in vivo* artifacts since fluorescent dyes persist in tissues after exosomes degradation. This is because lipid labeling is not exosomes specific and fluorescence might remain in degraded exosomes or other cellular structures, since they have an estimated half-life of several days [39]. Therefore, in long-term studies, the extended half-life of the lipophilic dye may result in the conservation of the fluorescent signal for longer than the exosomes persist itself, inducing false positive results as it was evaluated by Grange et al. in 2014 [40]. Ultimately, they confirmed that to reduce unspecific labeling, cells should be directly labeled with the dye, rather than exosomes. Exosomes could be then collected and further purified for administration [40].

5.3. Membrane permeable fluorescent dyes

Exosomes labeling can be achieved using membrane permeable chemical compounds. These dyes become confined to the cytosolic lumen and fluoresce as a consequence of esterification and include carboxyfluorescein succinimidyl ester (CFSE), 5(6)-carboxyfluorescein diacetate (CFDA) [41]. Another example is the use of calcein AM (an acetoxymethyl derivate of the fluorescent molecule calcein) that is a very good cytoplasmic fluorescent dye, since it attains high fluorescence intensities and exhibits an acceptable persistent labeling, given that it does not covalently link to intracellular molecules [33]. Calcein-labeling strategy is based on a membrane-permeant molecule that is nonfluorescent until it is activated by intra-vesicular enzymes [42]. Upon hydrolysis of the acetoxymethyl ester moieties by esterases, calcein becomes highly membrane impermeable [42]. The detection of calcein-labeled exosomes through flow cytometry has been already described and its use in some experiments has also been reported [43, 44].

Most of the studies performed to date include the use of membrane-labeled exosomes as described in the following examples. Sun et al., in 2010 administered i.p. fluorescent-labeled exosomes carrying curcumin (an anti-inflammatory agent), collected from EL-4 mouse lymphoma cells [15]. The exosomes accumulated in greater amounts in the liver, lungs, kidneys and spleen 1 h post-treatment. Interestingly, when exosomes were administered through the intranasal route, the distribution pattern was re-directed to the brain and intestines.

In 2011, Hood et al. demonstrated for the first time that exosomes isolated from melanoma cells supernatants induced LN conditioning *in vivo* [10]. DiR-labeled B16-F10 melanoma-derived exosomes were injected in the footpads of albino C57/BL6 mice and liposomes were used as control. Sentinel LN was harvested 48 h post-treatment, and fluorescent signals were evaluated using IVIS. They observed that melanoma exosomes home to the IN node ipsilateral to the injection site, whereas liposomes distributed equally in IN nodes both ipsilateral and contralateral to the site of injection. To assess how melanoma exosomes could influence free melanoma cells distribution within a lymphatic microenvironment during metastasis, three serial injections on the left footpad of mice were made in which the last one was accompanied with one million DiO labeled melanoma cells. Lymphatic distribution pattern of melanoma cells was assessed in the sentinel LN. An increased number of melanoma cells infiltrating located in the periphery of the node when mice were pre-treated with exosomes rather than liposomes. Furthermore, melanoma exosomes lead to an increased gene expression involved in cell recruitment, extracellular matrix remodeling and vascular proliferation factors contributing to a microenvironment within the sentinel nodes that favor melanoma cell homing, trapping and growth.

In 2012, Peinado et al. proposed a new role for melanoma-derived exosomes in which they educate bone marrow (BM) progenitor cells to acquire a pro-metastatic phenotype through MET signaling [8]. First, fluorescently labeled B16-F10 exosomes (using PKH67 dye) to analyze exosomes biodistribution were i.v. administered into naive mice. Exosomes were detected in the blood vessels and organs within 5 min after injection. Twenty-four hours post-treatment, exosomes were no longer found in blood circulation. Instead, exosomes were found in the major organotropic sites for B16-F10 metastasis including interstitium lungs, BM, liver and spleen. Next, B16-F10-derived exosomes were injected 3 times a week for 3 weeks, 7 days after orthotopically injection of B16-F10mCherry cells to assess melanoma-derived exosomes role in primary tumor growth and metastasis. Mice showed lung micro-metastasis at day 19 after tumor cell injection in contrast with the control (synthetic unilamellar liposomes). To evaluate the role of the metastatic potential of the cells of origin, equal amounts of exosomes from highly (B16-F10) or poorly (B16-F1) metastatic melanomas were i.v. injected into mice 3 times a week over 28 days, and then subcutaneously implanted B16-F10 cells expressing luciferase. Injection with B16-F10 exosomes resulted in a higher metastatic burden in the lungs and greater tissue distribution, including bone and brain when compared to mice injected with control particles or with B16-F1 exosomes. Notably, these observations indicate that exosomes content can mediate metastatic potential and organotropism. To further investigate this hypothesis and taking into consideration the central role of bone marrow-derived cells (BMDCs) in metastatic progression, they postulated whether tumor-derived exosomes could educate BMDCs and affect metastatic development. In a process, they termed bone marrow education, GFP-expressing mice were treated with B16-F10 exosomes 3 times a week for 28 days. Next, lethally irradiated mice were transplanted with the educated bone marrow and the mice were also subcutaneously injected with B16-F10 cells expressing mCherry. By pre-educating BMDCs with exosomes from a highly metastatic cancer cell line, an increase in the metastatic tumor burden and distribution in target tissues was observed, even for tumors with a low metastatic capacity. Overall, this work shows that by educating BMDCs tumor exosomes can regulate tumor metastasis. Further proteomics studies revealed MET as a potential candidate implicated in BM education given its previous described role in migration, invasion, angiogenesis and BM cells mobilization. Indeed, additional studies demonstrated that B16-F10-derived exosomes could transfer MET to BM progenitor cells, this way mediating pro-vasculogenic and metastatic effects (enhanced cell mobilization).

In 2015, Costa-Silva et al. proposed a mechanism in which pancreatic ductal adenocarcinoma (PDAC)-derived exosomes induce liver pre-metastatic niche formation in naive mice [11]. Authors demonstrated that Kupffer cells, macrophages present in the liver, uptake PDAC-derived exosomes, which activates the secretion of transforming growth factor β that in turn stimulates hepatic stellate cells to produce fibronectin. The resulting fibrotic microenvironment was showed to enhance the recruitment of BM-derived macrophages. Furthermore, macrophage migration inhibitory factor (MIF) was highly expressed in PDAC-derived exosomes, and its inhibition resulted in abrogation of liver pre-metastatic niche formation and metastasis. Collectively, these data suggest that PDAC-derived exosomal MIF primes the liver for metastasis.

In addition, Hoshino et al. took a step further in investigating pre-metastatic niche formation and unraveling exosomes organotropism [12]. The authors seek to demonstrate tumor-derived exosomes contribution to the establishment of a permissive microenvironment at future metastatic sites, describing their nonrandom biodistribution patterns. In all experiments performed, the authors use prepared pools of exosomes labeled with PKH dyes. They show that exosomes from mouse and human lung-, liver- and brain-tropic tumor cells fuse preferentially with resident cells at their predicted destination sites to prepare the pre-metastatic niche. Surprisingly, treatment with exosomes from lung-tropic tumor cells was sufficient to redirect the metastasis of bone-tropic tumor cells. Further exosomes proteomic studies revealed distinct integrin expression patterns that differed from tumor cells. They found that exosomes expressing integrin $\alpha v\beta 5$ specifically bind to Kupffer cells, mediating liver tropism, whereas exosomal integrins $\alpha 6\beta 4$ and $\alpha 6\beta 1$ mediated lung metastasis through binding with fibroblasts and epithelial cells. Moreover, when these integrins were blocked a decrease of exosomes uptake as well as metastasis formation was observed. Additionally, exosomes uptake by resident cells at metastatic sites mediated by the previously mentioned integrins was found to induce Src phosphorylation and activate the expression of pro-inflammatory S100 response. Altogether, these findings suggest that exosomal integrins are responsible for the adhesion of exosomes to target cells. Furthermore, this interaction activates, in the recipient cells, signaling pathways involved in inflammatory responses contributing to the formation of a microenvironment that supports the growth of metastatic cells.

Wen et al. associated exosomes derived from highly metastatic breast cancer cell lines with an increase in the metastatic potential partly due to an immune suppression of the tumor microenvironment [9]. Exosomes isolated from murine breast cancer cell lines (metastatic EO771 and 4T1, nonmetastatic 67NR) were labeled with DiD, a lipid-associating fluorescent dye and i.v. injected into mice. Exosomes biodistribution was evaluated in several organs 24 h post-injection using *in vivo* and *ex vivo* imaging and as control liposomes were used. Exogenously administered exosomes distributed mainly to the lungs irrespectively of the metastatic potential followed by spleen. Interestingly, lung and liver displayed higher signaling of exosomes derived from a nonmetastatic cell line compared to a highly metastatic one 4T1. In addition, regardless of the fact 4T1 breast cancer cells frequently exhibit liver tropism, its exosomes did not follow the same pattern. Additionally, exosomes derived from a nonmetastatic cell line distributed preferentially to the liver and lungs. Cumulatively, these results seem to point to the fact that exosomes not always follow the cells tropism patterns, which contrasts with the previously described findings made by Hoshino et al. Taken together, these data suggest that the biodistribution pattern of exosomes may be influenced by numerous factors including cell source, injection route and the amount administered. Therefore, the lack of well-established protocols to perform exosomes biodistribution studies may affect overall results. Nonetheless, Wen et al. further investigated which cell lineages were taking up exosomes in the lung and spleen. They found that around 14% and 3% of $CD45^+$ cells from the lung and spleen, respectively, were taking up EO771-derived exosomes. The majority were macrophages, $CD11b^+$ myeloid cells and dendritic cells. Nevertheless, this uptake pattern was similar in 4T1 and 67NR-derived exosomes. In addition, mice were injected *via* tail vein with a preparation of tumor-derived exosomes every three days for 30 days in order to evaluate the role of breast cancer-derived exosomes in pre-metastatic niche formation in an experiment similar to the one carried out by Peinado in 2012 [8]. They found that exosomes derived from highly metastatic breast cancer cells contributed to the establishment of a permissive microenvironment that in turn promoted cell metastasis trapping and growth in the lung and liver, which was not observed when using exosomes derived from nonmetastatic cells or liposomes. Moreover, EO771 exosomes accumulation in the lung was shown to promote an immunosuppressive microenvironment. This was observed through the recruitment of $CD11b^+/Ly6C^{med}$ granulocytic myeloid-derived suppressor cells, simultaneous to a decrease in T cell and natural killer cells frequency. Furthermore, EO771 exosomes treatment resulted in increased differentiation of naïve T cells ($CD44^{low}CD62L^{hi}$) to effector T cells ($CD44^{hi}CD62^{low}$). This phenomenon was previously described in other tumor microenvironments where T cells further differentiate into 'exhausted' T cells known to be nonfunctional and express high levels of immune inhibitory receptors contributing to cancer cells escape of the immune surveillance [45]. Wen et al. [9] demonstrated the immune suppressive potential of breast cancer-derived exosomes in promoting the pre-metastatic niche formation.

In 2014, Smyth et al. evaluated the tissue distribution of exosomes derived from breast and prostate cancer cell lines when i.v. administered into healthy or tumor-bearing mice [46]. Exosomes were isolated from cell culture supernatants of 4T1, PC3 and MCF-7 cells. Mice were inoculated with 4T1 cells in the mammary fat pad (MFP) and 15 days after inoculation they were i.v. injected *via* tail vein with 4T1 exosomes fluorescently labeled with DiR. *In vivo* imaging was performed using IVIS at 1, 8 and 24 h post-injection. At the 24-h time point, mice were sacrificed and organs excised for *ex vivo* imaging. One hour after treatment exosomes distributed primarily to the liver and spleen. To further investigate exosomes biodistribution, PC3 and MCF-7 exosomes were radiolabeled with indium-111 and injected i.v. into nude mice-bearing PC3 tumors or nontumor-bearing nude mice. Blood clearance analysis revealed that 3-h post-injection less than 5% of the injected vesicles remained in circulation. Furthermore, the presence of the tumor did not affect exosomes blood clearance. Overall, biodistribution patterns were analyzed 24 h after treatment and found to be very similar to the 4T1 experiment, with greater accumulation in the liver and spleen, followed by the kidneys when compared to other organs including PC3 tumors. In addition, the biodistribution pattern of PC3 exosomes was basically the same in PC3 tumor-bearing nude mice or nontumor-bearing mice. Next, the authors wanted to assess the influence of the innate immune system on exosomes biodistribution and clearance in tumor-bearing mice. Therefore, they inoculated 4T1 cells in the MFP of Balb/c, nude and NOD.CB17-Prkdcscid/J mice and i.v.-injected 4T1 exosomes. It is important to take into consideration that nude mice suffer from a lack of adaptive immune response, while NOD.CB17-Prkdcscid/J mice suffer from impaired innate immunity including impaired complement activity. 4T1 exosomes in nude and Balb/c mice distributed preferentially to the liver and spleen after 20 min post-injection, with levels remaining unaltered over the course of 2 h, suggesting that the adaptive immune system is not responsible for the clearance of exosomes. Interestingly, NOD.CB17-Prkdcscid/J mice displayed an increase in the accumulation of 4T1 exosomes in the liver and spleen between 20 min and 2 h post-injection. The slower uptake of exosomes by the reticuloendothelial system (RES) in NOD.CB17-Prkdcscid/J mice suggests that the innate immune system, alongside with complement opsonization, contributes to exosomes blood clearance.

Recently, Wiklander et al. established a set of experiments demonstrating that EVs biodistribution is dependent on many factors, including cell source, exosomes concentration and route of administration [13]. They injected 1×10^{10} particles/gram body weight (p/g) *via* tail vein of DiR-labeled EVs isolated from HEK293T cell culture supernatant. To assess their biodistribution, organs were harvested for *ex vivo* imaging 24 h post-injection. Importantly, they performed perfused and nonperfused conditions prior to organs harvesting to confirm whether signaling was coming from organs or was due to the presence of labeled EVs in circulation. In addition, EV-free medium was subject to the same protocol as for EV-DiR labeled to exclude the possibility of monitoring free dye. Interestingly, perfusion did not seem to affect EVs biodistribution and EV-free medium injection resulted in insignificant signal in all organs. EVs derived from HEK293T expressing CD63-EGFP plasmid were also used at a concentration of 2.9×10^{10} (p/g). Twenty-four hours post-injection organs were harvested and analyzed. Signal was found on the parenchyma of the liver and spleen. However, little or no signal was detected in lungs and kidney. Next, they evaluated whether EV biodistribution was EV dose dependent. Therefore, they injected different amounts of DiR-labeled HEK293T EVs (0.25×10^{10}, 1×10^{10} and 1.5×10^{10}). Indeed, a positive correlation between EV dosage and total tissue fluorescence was observed. In addition to this phenomenon, a shift of the relative distribution of EVs among organs also occurred. Relative liver accumulation decreased sequentially with the initial amount of EVs injected. The authors hypothesized that this decrease could result from the saturation of the mononuclear phagocyte system/RES allowing a more effective evasion of the liver at higher amounts. Since the use of lipophilic dyes is associated with prolonged half-life when compared to the EV, the authors evaluated DiR-labeled HEK293T EVs biodistribution at different time points. EVs distribution pattern kept unchanged during 24-h post-injection. However, major differences registered at the time point of 48 h. Fluorescence signal decreased in heart, gastro-intestinal (GI)-tract and kidneys, while the signal in the pancreas suffered a significant increase. These alterations can be due to a re-distribution of EVs or artifacts, since fluorescence dyes are known to have half-lives of several days. In addition, Wiklander et al. evaluated the distribution outcome when the EVs were administered through different routes. In all cases, 1×10^{10} p/g DiR-labeled EV were injected *via* i.v., i.p. or s.c. Interestingly, the different injection routes were associated with different distribution patterns. I.p. and s.c. injections lead to lower EVs accumulation in the liver and spleen, while increased accumulation was detected in the pancreas and GI tract, contrarily to what it was observed for the i.v. injections. Moreover, i.p. injections resulted in higher total tissue fluorescence, while s.c. injections resulted in the lowest one. Their careful analyses also included the influence of the cell of origin in biodistribution outcomes. Three mouse cell sources were used: a muscle cell line C2C12, a melanoma cell line B16F10 and a primary immature BM-derived dendritic cells (DC). Additionally, xenotransplantation of EVs from rat cells—oligodendrocytes OLN-93—and from cells of human origin—HEK293T and primary human mesenchymal stromal cells (MSC)—were used for cross-species studies. All experiments were performed using 1×10^{10} p/g DiR-labeled-EV administered *via* i.v.. Overall, the distribution pattern from the different mouse cell sources did not vary much with spleen, liver, GI tract and lungs being the greatest accumulation sites. Nevertheless, some significant differences were encountered. For instance, C2C12-derived EVs were highly present at the liver, while in the lung displayed the lowest amount of signal accumulated. B16F10 derived EVs were in turn most frequently accumulated in the GI tract, and DC-derived EVs were highly accumulated in the spleen when compared to the other mouse cell sources. Notably, *in vivo* biodistribution patterns did not differ when xenotransplanted EVs were used. MSC-derived EVs displayed higher accumulation in the liver, while the GI tract was the lowest compared to EVs derived from HEK293T and OLN-93 cells. Interestingly, HEK293T, OLN-93 and C2C12 derived EVs presented similar tissue distribution outcomes suggesting that species of origins does not seem to affect the patterns observed. Finally, HEK293T-derived EVs were found to accumulate greatly in the liver and spleen in B16F10 tumor-bearing mice, 24 h post-injection with 1×10^{10} p/g DiR-labeled EV administered *via* i.v., with only 3% of the total fluorescence being detected in the tumor. Wicklander elegantly showed for the first time the different confounders added to EVs *in vivo* biodistribution studies, highlighting the urgency to develop new reliable models.

Another method consists on the genetic engineering of cells to direct the expression of fluorescent markers to the exosomal membrane resulting in labeled exosomes production. Exosomes can be isolated from these cells culture supernatants or cells can be directly injected into mice. One commonly used example is the GFP-CD63 construct. The CD63 is a tetraspanin, a membrane-associated protein and is known as a general marker of exosomes [47]. Suetsugu and collaborators were one of the first ones to orthotopically inject stable expressing GFP-tagged CD63 cells [48]. They demonstrated that tumor-derived exosomes serve as a central mediators for communication not only between cancer cells but also with their microenvironment components. They produced mouse breast cancer cells (MMT) and human breast cancer cells (MDA-MD-231) RFP labeled stably expressing GFP-tagged CD63 (MMT-RFP/GFP-Exo and MDA-MD-231-RFP/GFP-Exo, respectively). Hence, cells were red and producing green exosomes. To generate orthotopic mouse models of breast cancer metastasis to the lung, they orthotopically injected MMT-RFP/GFP-Exo or MDA-MD-231-RFP/GFP-Exo cells into the MFP of nude mice. Overall, using confocal laser scan microscopy (CLSM), they observed that both in primary tumors and in lung metastasis breast cancer cells secreted exosomes into the tumor microenvironment. To confirm GFP exosomes integration in mice host cells, RFP nude mice were orthotopically injected with the cells previously mentioned into the MFP. GFP-labeled exosomes were taken up by stromal cells namely fibroblasts. Finally, blood samples analysis by CLSM confirmed the presence of GFP exosomes in circulation of mice-bearing lung metastasis.

Nonetheless, when designing these fusion plasmids, one should consider the influence they may have in the protein normal functions. Interestingly, it has been shown that GFP fusion to the N- or C-terminus of CD63 influences protein distribution in rat basophilic leukemia (RBL) cells [49]. When GFP was linked to the C-terminus of CD63 (CD63-GFP), the fused proteins were expressed on both the granule membranes and plasma membranes of RBL cells as native CD63 proteins. Contrarily, when the GFP was conjugated to the N-terminus of CD63 (GFP-CD63), it was homogeneously distributed in the cytoplasm, not being present on granules or the plasma membrane [49]. These results suggested the possibility that the N-terminus of CD63 might play an important role in the establishment of protein localization.

Other approaches developed by Lai et al. in 2014 included a multiplex reporter system consisting of enhanced (EGFP) and tandem dimer tomato (tdTomato) fluorescent proteins fused at NH2-termini with specific palmitoylation signals, enabling EV membrane labeling [39]. By treating cells with EVs carrying fluorescently labeled siRNA, they observed EVs uptake in donor cells. Notably, by combining fluorescent and bioluminescent EVs membrane reporters, they elegantly demonstrated EVs uptake and translation of nascent EV-derived cargo mRNAs in cancer cells *in vitro* as early as 1 h after exposing cells to EVs.

Recently, a new approach was put forward that allows the study of the function of transfer of EVs *in vitro* and *in vivo* settings without the requirement to artificially expose cells to isolated and concentrated pools of EVs [50]. To study the exchange of EVs, the Cre-loxP system was used to fluorescently label Cre-reporter cells that take up the EVs released from cells that express Cre recombinase. Donor cells expressing Cre recombinase were CFP positive (blue), whereas unrecombined Cre-reporter cells were DsRed positive (red) and those that have internalized the EV and have recombined switch from red to green. They demonstrated that the switch in color was due to Cre mRNA containing EVs and not by other mechanisms including free Cre mRNA or protein. Using this technology, they were able to assess whether different types of nontumor cells take up tumor-released EVs [51]. Cre-expressing B16 melanoma cells were injected into mice ubiquitously expressing the Cre-LoxP reporter tdTomato (tdTomato B6 mice). Notably, nontumor cells expressing tdTomato were found in all analyzed tissues (tumors, lymph nodes, lungs and spleens). This pool of cells presented either $CD45^-$ or $CD45^+$ cells (a general immune cell marker), suggesting that both non-immune cells and immune cells took up tumor-released EVs. By immunohistochemistry, they found that some of those cells were neutrophils and macrophages using different markers. Therefore, authors concluded that tumor cell-derived EVs are taken up by both tumor cells and different sorts of nontumor cells. They next assessed if tumor cells could uptake EVs released from nontumor cells. B16 melanoma cells that express the Cre-LoxP reporter were injected into B6 mice that ubiquitously expressed Cre. Interestingly, tumor cells with changed phenotype due to the uptake of Cre derived from EVs released from nontumor cells were found sporadically. Therefore, B16 melanoma cells render the ability to take up EVs from healthy cells; however, this transfer does not seem to happen in the same extent as the opposite does. Further studies demonstrated that less malignant tumor cells located either in the same or within distant tumors took up EVs released by tumor cells. In addition, gene expression arrays lead to the discovery of a differential mRNA profile with a significant enrichment of mRNA molecules involved in migration and metastasis in EVs compared to the cells, both of which promote tumor progression. Overall, data suggest that malignant tumor cells, through transfer of EVs, increase migration and metastatic capacity of less malignant cells *in vivo*. Importantly, it was the first time that the transfer of functional cargo through EVs was shown *in vivo*, demonstrating their biological role. This approach is versatile once it can be used in nearly all cell types and more importantly the *in vivo* application allows to study the exchange of EVs in a more natural context, one where cells interact and respond to multiple stimulus of different cell types [50]. Nevertheless, this new strategy is not exosomes specific. Therefore, an *in vivo* model that presents itself as closer to the normal biological system, enabling the study of exosomes natural fate and biological function is still missing.

6. Concluding remarks

Collectively, exosomes spatiotemporal distribution is still elusive, mostly because *in vivo* exosomes research relies on their purification from cells in culture and *in vitro* treatment of other cultured cells or *in vivo* administration in tumor-bearing mice. Despite latest findings, results from *in vitro* experiments cannot be directly extrapolated to the *in vivo* context and need to be carefully analyzed, as clearly pointed by Zomer et al. [50]. Thus far this artificial approach has not given us insight of the actual communication routes of exosomes in the organism, highlighting the great demand for improved animal models that allow exosomes studies *in vivo*. Genetically engineered mouse models (GEMM) could be a promising approach to address the current technical limitations faced. Ideally, these models should allow tracing tumor-derived exosomes while retaining the animal immune system. This important modulator of tumor development is most of the times inexistent since the majority of the experiments are performed using immune deficient mice. Exosomes derived both from tumor and normal cells are known to modulate the immune response as well as the cellular physiology in the tumor surroundings, contributing to a favorable and permissive microenvironment for the establishment of the tumor and potentially spread to other parts of the organism [52, 53]. It would be very useful to track tumor-derived exosomes in a well-established cancer GEMM model by using an exosomes marker that is fused to a fluorescent protein. Since GFP, RFP and CFP transgenic nude mice appear to have a life span similar to that of non-transgenic nude mice, fluorescent proteins are considered nontoxic and are a promising method for *in vivo* imaging [54]. The scientific community would greatly benefit from these animal models that mimic the best way possible the natural physiology of such a complex disease. Despite intensive efforts, many questions remain unanswered in the field of extracellular vesicles, which the answer could revolutionize today's view both of the normal organism physiology as well as in a cancer context.

Acknowledgements

SAM laboratory is supported by the project NORTE-01-0145-FEDER-000029, supported by Norte Portugal Regional Programme (NORTE 2020), under the PORTUGAL 2020 Partnership Agreement, through the European Regional Development Fund (ERDF) and FEDER funds through the COMPETE Program (POCI-01/0145-FEDER-016618), national funds from FCT – Foundation for Science and Technology PTDC/BIM-ONC/2754/2014 and Maratonas da Saúde. SAM is supported by FCT – Foundation for Science and Technology (IF/00543/2013). We thank Dr. Nuno Barros for the help with the design of the figures included in this chapter.

Author details

Bárbara Adem[1,2] and Sónia A. Melo[1,2,3*]

*Address all correspondence to: smelo@ipatimup.pt

1 Institute for Research and Innovation in Health (i3S), University of Porto, Portugal, Porto, Portugal

2 Institute of Molecular Pathology & Immunology of the University of Porto (IPATIMUP), Porto, Portugal

3 Medical Faculty of the University of Porto, Porto, Portugal

References

[1] Kalluri R. The biology and function of exosomes in cancer. The Journal of Clinical Investigation. 2016;**126**(4):1208-1215

[2] Colombo M, Raposo G, Thery C. Biogenesis, secretion, and intercellular interactions of exosomes and other extracellular vesicles. Annual Review of Cell and Developmental Biology 2014;**30**:255-289

[3] Yang S, et al. Detection of mutant KRAS and TP53 DNA in circulating exosomes from healthy individuals and patients with pancreatic cancer. Cancer Biology & Therapy. 2017

[4] Skog J, et al. Glioblastoma microvesicles transport RNA and proteins that promote tumour growth and provide diagnostic biomarkers. Nature Cell Biology. 2008;**10**(12):1470-1476

[5] Valadi H, et al. Exosome-mediated transfer of mRNAs and microRNAs is a novel mechanism of genetic exchange between cells. Nature Cell Biology. 2007;**9**(6):654-659

[6] Melo SA, et al. Cancer exosomes perform cell-independent microRNA biogenesis and promote tumorigenesis. Cancer Cell. 2014;**26**(5):707-721

[7] Baglio SR, et al. Blocking tumor-educated MSC paracrine activity halts osteosarcoma progression. Clinical Cancer Research. 2017. [Epub ahead of print]

[8] Peinado H, et al. Melanoma exosomes educate bone marrow progenitor cells toward a pro-metastatic phenotype through MET. Nature Medicine. 2012;**18**(6):883-891

[9] Wen SW, et al. The biodistribution and immune suppressive effects of breast cancer–derived exosomes. Cancer Research. 2016;**76**(23):6816

[10] Hood JL, San RS, Wickline SA. Exosomes released by melanoma cells prepare sentinel lymph nodes for tumor metastasis. Cancer Research. 2011;**71**(11):3792

[11] Costa-Silva B, et al. Pancreatic cancer exosomes initiate pre-metastatic niche formation in the liver. Nature Cell Biology. 2015;**17**(6):816-826

[12] Hoshino A, et al. Tumour exosome integrins determine organotropic metastasis. Nature. 2015;**527**(7578):329-335

[13] Wiklander OPB, et al. Extracellular vesicle in vivo biodistribution is determined by cell source, route of administration and targeting. Journal of Extracellular Vesicles. 2015;**4**(1)

[14] Lai CP, et al. Dynamic biodistribution of extracellular vesicles in vivo using a multimodal imaging reporter. ACS Nano. 2014;**8**(1):483-494

[15] Sun D, et al. A novel nanoparticle drug delivery system: The anti-inflammatory activity of curcumin is enhanced when encapsulated in exosomes. Molecular Therapy. 2010;**18**(9):1606-1614

[16] Takahashi Y, et al. Visualization and in vivo tracking of the exosomes of murine melanoma B16-BL6 cells in mice after intravenous injection. Journal of Biotechnology. 2013; **165**(2):77-84

[17] Santos EB, et al. Sensitive in vivo imaging of T cells using a membrane-bound Gaussia princeps luciferase. Nature Medicine. 2009;**15**(3):338-344

[18] Delcayre A, et al. Exosome display technology: Applications to the development of new diagnostics and therapeutics. Blood Cells, Molecules, and Diseases 2005;**35**(2):158-168

[19] Imai T, et al. Macrophage-dependent clearance of systemically administered B16BL6-derived exosomes from the blood circulation in mice. Journal of Extracellular Vesicles. 2015;**4**:26238. DOI:10.3402/jev.v4.26238

[20] Morishita M, et al. Quantitative analysis of tissue distribution of the B16BL6-derived exosomes using a streptavidin-lactadherin fusion protein and iodine-125-labeled biotin derivative after intravenous injection in mice. Journal of Pharmaceutical Sciences. 2015;**104**(2):705-713

[21] Hwang DW, et al. Noninvasive imaging of radiolabeled exosome-mimetic nanovesicle using 99mTc-HMPAO. Scientific Reports 2015,**5**:15636

[22] Phillips WT, Goins BA, Bao A. Radioactive liposomes. Wiley Interdisciplinary Reviews. Nanomedicine and Nanobiotechnology. 2009;**1**(1):69-83

[23] Jang SC, et al. Bioinspired exosome-mimetic nanovesicles for targeted delivery of chemotherapeutics to malignant tumors. ACS Nano. 2013;**7**(9):7698-7710

[24] Varga Z, et al. Radiolabeling of extracellular vesicles with (99m)Tc for quantitative in vivo imaging studies. Cancer Biotherapy and Radiopharmaceuticals. 2016;**31**(5):168-173

[25] Egli A, et al. Organometallic 99mTc-aquaion labels peptide to an unprecedented high specific activity. Journal of Nuclear Medicine. 1999;**40**(11):1913-1917

[26] Hu L, Wickline SA, Hood JL. Magnetic resonance imaging of melanoma exosomes in lymph nodes. Magnetic Resonance in Medicine. 2015;**74**(1):266-271

[27] Busato A, et al. Magnetic resonance imaging of ultrasmall superparamagnetic iron oxide-labeled exosomes from stem cells: A new method to obtain labeled exosomes. International Journal of Nanomedicine 2016;**11**:2481-2490

[28] Bull E, et al. Stem cell tracking using iron oxide nanoparticles. International Journal of Nanomedicine 2014;**9**:1641-1653

[29] Alam SR, et al. Vascular and plaque imaging with ultrasmall superparamagnetic particles of iron oxide. Journal of Cardiovascular Magnetic Resonance. 2015;**17**(1):83

[30] Malatesta M, et al. Diaminobenzidine photoconversion is a suitable tool for tracking the intracellular location of fluorescently labelled nanoparticles at transmission electron microscopy. European Journal of Histochemistry : EJH. 2012;**56**:e20. DOI: 10.4081/ejh.2012.20

[31] Kahlert C, et al. Identification of double stranded genomic DNA spanning all chromosomes with mutated KRAS and p53 DNA in the serum exosomes 7of patients with pancreatic cancer. Journal of Biological Chemistry. 2014;**289**(7):3869-75

[32] Ullal AJ, Pisetsky DS, Reich CF, 3rd. Use of SYTO 13, a fluorescent dye binding nucleic acids, for the detection of microparticles in in vitro systems. Cytometry. Part A. 2010; **77**(3):294-301

[33] Parish CR, Fluorescent dyes for lymphocyte migration and proliferation studies. Immunology and Cell Biology. 1999;**77**(6):499-508

[34] Alvarez-Erviti L, et al. Delivery of siRNA to the mouse brain by systemic injection of targeted exosomes. Nature Biotechnology. 2011;**29**(4):341-345

[35] Zech D, et al. Tumor-exosomes and leukocyte activation: An ambivalent crosstalk. Cell Communication and Signaling. 2012;**10**(1):37

[36] Tian T, et al. Dynamics of exosome internalization and trafficking. Journal of Cellular Physiology. 2013;**228**(7):1487-1495

[37] Tian T, et al. Visualizing of the cellular uptake and intracellular trafficking of exosomes by live-cell microscopy. Journal of Cellular Biochemistry. 2010;**111**(2):488-496

[38] Di Rocco G, Baldari S, Toietta G. Towards therapeutic delivery of extracellular vesicles: Strategies for in vivo tracking and biodistribution analysis. Stem Cells International 2016;**2016**:12

[39] Lai CP, et al. Visualization and tracking of tumour extracellular vesicle delivery and RNA translation using multiplexed reporters. Nature Communications. 2015;**6**:7029

[40] Grange C, et al. Biodistribution of mesenchymal stem cell-derived extracellular vesicles in a model of acute kidney injury monitored by optical imaging. International Journal of Molecular Medicine. 2014;**33**(5):1055-1063

[41] Temchura VV, et al. Enhancement of immunostimulatory properties of exosomal vaccines by incorporation of fusion-competent G protein of vesicular stomatitis virus. Vaccine. 2008;**26**(29-30):3662-3672

[42] Gray WD, Mitchell AJ, Searles CD. An accurate, precise method for general labeling of extracellular vesicles. MethodsX. 2015;**2**:360-367

[43] Gray WD, et al. Identification of therapeutic covariant microRNA clusters in hypoxia-treated cardiac progenitor cell exosomes using systems biology. Circulation Research. 2015;**116**(2):255

[44] Mitchell PJ, et al. Can urinary exosomes act as treatment response markers in prostate cancer? Journal of Translational Medicine. 2009;**7**(1):4

[45] Jiang Y, Li Y, Zhu B. T-cell exhaustion in the tumor microenvironment. Cell Death & Disease. 2015;**6**(6):e1792

[46] Smyth T, et al. Biodistribution and delivery efficiency of unmodified tumor-derived exosomes. Journal of Controlled Release: Official Journal of the Controlled Release Society. 2015;**199**:145-155

[47] Andreu Z, Yáñez-Mó M. Tetraspanins in extracellular vesicle formation and function. Frontiers in Immunology 2014;**5**:442

[48] Suetsugu A, et al. Imaging exosome transfer from breast cancer cells to stroma at metastatic sites in orthotopic nude-mouse models. Advanced Drug Delivery Reviews. 2013;**65**(3):383-390

[49] Amano T, et al. Dynamics of intracellular granules with CD63-GFP in rat basophilic leukemia cells. Journal of Biochemistry. 2001;**129**(5):739-744

[50] Zomer A, et al. Studying extracellular vesicle transfer by a Cre-loxP method. Nature Protocols. 2016;**11**(1):87-101

[51] Zomer A, et al. In vivo imaging reveals extracellular vesicle-mediated phenocopying of metastatic behavior. Cell. 2015;**161**(5):1046-1057

[52] Webber J, et al. Cancer exosomes trigger fibroblast to myofibroblast differentiation. Cancer Research. 2010;**70**(23):9621

[53] Thery C, Ostrowski M, Segura E. Membrane vesicles as conveyors of immune responses. Nature Reviews. Immunology. 2009;**9**(8):581-593

[54] Hoffman RM. Application of GFP imaging in cancer. Laboratory Investigation; A Journal of Technical Methods and Pathology. 2015;**95**(4):432-452

Section 2

Exosome in Viral Infection

Chapter 4

Exosomes and Their Role in Viral Infections

Gulfaraz Khan, Waqar Ahmed and Pretty S. Philip

Additional information is available at the end of the chapter

http://dx.doi.org/10.5772/intechopen.69397

Abstract

Exosomes are excretory nano-vesicles that are formed by the cell's endocytic system and shed from the surface of almost all types of cells. These tiny extracellular vesicles, once thought to be "garbage bags for cells," carry a wide variety of molecules of cellular origin, including proteins, lipids, and RNAs, that are selectively incorporated during the formation of exosomes. Exosomes are now known to play a central role in several important biological processes such as cellular communication, intercellular transfer of bioactive molecules, and immune modulation. Recent advances in the field have shown that a number of animal viruses can exploit the exosomal pathway by incorporating specific cellular or viral factors within exosomes, in order to modulate the cellular microenvironment and influence downstream processes such as host immunity and virus spread. In this chapter, we provide an overview of our current understanding of exosome biogenesis and how this normal physiological process is hijacked by some pathogenic viruses. Viral components that appear to be selectively incorporated into exosomes and the potential role of these exosomes in viral pathogenesis are discussed. Identifying viral signatures in exosomes and their mode of action is fundamental for any future diagnostic and therapeutic strategies for viral infections.

Keywords: exosomes, viruses, immune modulation, pathogenesis, biomarkers

1. Introduction

Exosomes are nano-secretory vesicles ranging in size from 30 to 100 nm and having a density between 1.13 and 1.19 g/ml [1]. Exosomes are derived from the cell's endosomal pathway, and their membranes are rich in lipids such as sphingolipids, ceramide, and cholesterol [2]. These tiny vesicles are released by virtually all cell types, but at varying degree, upon fusion of multivesicular bodies (MVBs) with the plasma membrane [3–5]. It is now well established that exosomes are not the cell's trash bags, as initially thought, but rather they serve as important nano-vehicles for the transport of specific cargo in and out of the cells [6]. Depending on their cargo, exosomes can mediate certain intercellular communication processes [7, 8]. Although the mechanism of how this cargo is selected for packaging into these vesicles destined for excretion remains poorly understood, it is believed that the endosomal membranes play a central role in this process [9, 10].

A number of molecular mechanisms are involved in the formation of intraluminal vesicles (ILVs) and multivesicular bodies (MVBs) in a cell. One of the best studied and well-characterized group of proteins involved in this process belong to the ESCRT (endosomal sorting complex required for transport) family of proteins [11–13]. These proteins are believed to play a role in the inward budding and scission of ILVs. One of the mechanism by which viruses hijack the exosome pathway is by directly interfering with the machinery involved in exosome biogenesis, such as the ESCRT proteins [14]. Others such as the oligomerization of the tetraspanin complexes [15], the sphingomyelinase pathways [16], phospholipase D2, and ADP ribosylation factor-6–mediated pathways have also been reported to be involved in the ILV budding process [17]. Another family of proteins that are essential for vesicular formation, trafficking, and fusion in eukaryotic cells belongs to a large family of highly conserved proteins known as Rab GTPases [18]. A number of Rab proteins such as Rab5 and Rab7 have been shown to be important in endosome maturation and sorting of material in the ILVs [19, 20]. Rab27 a/b are involved in the fusion of the ILVs with the plasma membrane and release of exosomes [50]. A number of other Rab GTPases are also found to play an instrumental role in exosome release. Depending on the cell type, Rab5, Rab7, Rab11, Rab27, and Rab35 have all been implicated in the release of vesicles. Altering the levels of any of these Rabs may lead to interference with progression of exosomal cargo at specific endocytic locations [20]. The fact that the exosomal pathway has some similarities with certain phases of viral life cycle has led to the observations that a number of viruses can indeed hijack the exosome pathway during their replication and pathogenesis [21, 22].

2. Viruses and the exosomal pathway

The endocytic pathway and the budding of viruses, especially enveloped viruses, share many common features. Both processes require generation of membrane curving, packaging of specific cargo, and membrane budding for release from the cell [22]. What is most surprising is that different viruses with very different evolutionary paths appear to converge in their use of the host endocytic pathway in the entry and exit from their host cells [23]. The receptor or clathrin-mediated endocytosis to enter the cell is found to be utilized by a number of viruses of the Flaviviridae family, which includes medically important pathogens such as hepatitis C (HCV), West Nile (WNV), Dengue, and Zika viruses [24–27]. These viruses can enter the late endosomes and then fuse with the ILVs within the endosome compartments [28]. Recently, it was shown that HCV can incorporate its full-length RNA genome into the ILVs and be excreted out via exosomes, and retain infectivity [29, 30]. Since HCV is fairly small, it is possible that HCV infectious particles could be released directly within exosomes and account for infection. However, the observation that exosomes isolated from

HCV sub-genomic replicon cell lines lacking HCV structural proteins remained infectious argues against the notion that mature viral particles are released in exosomes [30]. Currently, HCV and hepatitis A virus (HAV) are the only viruses that have been shown to incorporate their full-length genomic RNA within exosomes [31]. Another virus that can utilize the endosomal/exosomal system to deliver viral cargo to uninfected cells is the human immunodeficiency virus (HIV-1). Based on the similarities between HIV-1 assembly and egress, and exosome biogenesis, Gould et al. proposed the "Trojan exosome hypothesis," in which they suggested that HIV has evolved to exploit the exosome system to infect cells in the absence of the receptor-mediated interaction [32, 33]. This hypothesis is supported by the observation that HIV virions are released together with exosomes, but the infectivity is reduced in the absence of exosomes, implying that the process of exosome release from HIV-infected cells probably also contributes to the release of HIV virions. This mechanism was demonstrated using HIV-infected dendritic cells, which were able to transfer the virus to closely associated uninfected T cells via exosomes [34, 35]. Unlike HCV, direct packaging of HIV genomic RNA into exosomes has not been observed, probably reflecting the findings that HIV predominately buds from the plasma membrane and not from the endosomal pathway [36–38].

2.1. Viruses hijack the ESCRT and Rab GTPases involved in exosome biogenesis

Viruses are obligate intracellular parasites that hijack cellular pathways to complete their life cycle. In recent years, an accumulating body of data has emerged suggesting that some viruses can also manipulate with the vesicular trafficking machinery for their assembly, egress, and transmission [39, 40]. For example, HIV has been shown to exploit the ESCRT, lipid raft domains, and Rab GTPases components, all of which are involved in exosome biogenesis [23, 41, 42]. Specifically, HIV Gag has been shown to interact with exosomal tetraspanins, especially CD63 and CD81, to aid in virion egress [42]. Using electron microscopy, human herpesvirus 6 (HHV-6) virions have been shown to be present in MVBs and egress together with exosomes through the same pathway [43]. HHV-6 infection dramatically increases MVB formation, suggesting that the endosomal pathway is likely to be important for HHV-6 infection and assembly [43]. Furthermore, HHV-6 glycoprotein gB was found to co-localize with CD63 [43], but the importance of this association for virus egress remains to be demonstrated. Besides interfering with the ESCRT pathway, some viruses can also utilize the Rab GTPase complexes to assist in their replication and egress processes. Several negative strand RNA viruses, such as influenza A virus (IAV), hantavirus, and respiratory syncytial virus (RSV), have all been reported to utilize the Rab pathway for their transport to the plasma membrane for exit [44–47]. It is known that interfering with Rab11 levels can inhibit or promote the release of exosome-containing contents such as transferrin, HSP-70, flotillin, and anthrax toxin [44, 48, 49]. In the case of hantavirus-infected cells, depletion of Rab11 results in a tenfold reduction in virion production [46]. Similarly, IAV and RSV also appear to hijack the Rab11 pathway to their benefit [45, 47]. Rab27a, another member of the Rab GTPase family, has also been shown to be essential for exosome biogenesis, particularly in the steps involving the fusion of MVBs with plasma membrane for the final release of exosomes [50, 51]. For example, in cytomegalovirus (CMV)-infected cells, the levels of Rab27a are increased and co-localized with the viral envelope components at assembly sites in the cytoplasm [52], but the molecular mechanisms and ultimate changes to exosome production remain to be elucidated. HIV proteins are also found to interact with Rab27a resulting in increased levels of exosome formation [41, 53]. Herpes simplex virus 1 (HSV-1) is another virus that appears to use Rab27a for its intracellular transport and exocytosis [54, 55]. Depletion or down-regulation of Rab27a leads to decrease in HSV-1 viral production [54, 55].

The regulatory functions of the Rab GTPase mentioned above are still not fully understood. However, it is widely accepted that cells react to stimuli to adjust the distribution and levels of intracellular proteins as well as their degradation, secretion, and recycling [56]. Manipulation of specific steps in the endocytic pathway by viruses highlights the need for further research to unravel the complex interplay between regulators of the endocytic process and exosome release. Such studies may shed light to potential targets for anti-virals.

2.2. Viral signatures in exosomes

The discovery that certain features in the life cycle of viruses and the cellular endosomal/exosomal pathway are common, and that some viruses can exploit the exosomal pathway to their benefit, triggered a search to identify viral signatures in exosomes. This line of research has obvious downstream benefits, not only in terms of viral diagnosis, but also for understanding the mechanisms of viral-mediated pathogenesis. We now have a growing list of viral-specific components that have been identified in exosomes (**Table 1**). Moreover, functional analysis of excreted exosomes carrying viral components is beginning to shed light on how some viruses can modulate cellular processes as diverse as immune evasion, apoptosis, proliferation, and even viral infectivity (**Table 1**). In this context, one family of viruses that has been widely studied is the human herpesviruses. This family of viruses contains two members, namely Epstein-Barr virus (EBV) and Kaposi's sarcoma virus (KSV), that are oncogenic and implicated in the pathogenesis of a number of human malignancies [57]. Both of these viruses have now been shown to exploit the exosome pathway to secrete various components ranging from proteins to various species of RNAs, including messenger RNAs (mRNA), microRNAs (miRNA), and small non-protein coding RNAs [58–61]. In fact, viral miRNAs (vmiRNA) were first identified in EBV-infected cells [62] and subsequently shown to be excreted out of cells via exosomes [63]. It is now known that exosomes shed from EBV-infected cells contain a large number of viral miRNAs, most of which appear to be smaller products of larger BamH1 EBV transcripts [64, 65]. It is believed that these viral miRNAs, together with cellular miRNAs, play a role in modulating the expression of target genes in recipient cells (**Figure 1**) [59, 65–67]. Recently, it was shown that the two non-protein coding EBV small RNAs, EBER-1 and EBER-2, are also consistently excreted from infected cells within exosomes [68]. EBERs are highly abundant EBV RNA polymerase II/III transcripts expressed in all EBV latently infected cells. The significance of their high abundance within infected cells, or the reasons for their release in exosomes, remains intriguing. One study showed that EBERs released from infected cells could induce innate immune responses via activation of Toll-like receptor 3-mediated signaling [69]. In addition to RNAs, a number of studies have shown that EBV-infected cells can also excrete viral-specific proteins, including the latent membrane protein 1 and 2A (LMP-1, LMP-2A) and the viral envelop glycoprotein 350 (gp350) [70–73]. Export of these proteins via exosomes indicates another dimension to how EBV can modulate cellular processes, not only within the cells it infects, but also in the surrounding cells.

Virus	Main cellular target	Viral cargo reported in exosomes	Potential effect of viral exosomes	References
EBV	Lymphocytes	LMP1, 2A, gp350, vmiRNA, EBERs, vRNA	Proliferation, apoptosis, immune evasion, viral reactivation	[63, 68, 70, 72, 73, 92]
HSV-1	Epithelial cells	VP16, HSV gB, ICP 127, vmiRNA	Increase infectivity, viral spread, and latency	[116, 128]
CMV	WBC, epithelial cells	CMV gB	Infection of myeloid dendritic cells, increased viral infectivity	[129]
HHV-8	WBC, endothelial cells	vmiRNA, vRNA	Immune modulation, cell metabolism	[60, 61]
HIV-1	Lymphocytes	vmiRTAR, vmiRNA, Nef	Inhibition of apoptosis, stimulate proinflammatory cytokines, down-regulation of CD4 and MHC I, increased susceptibility of naïve T cells, antiviral activity	[81, 82, 130, 131]
HTLV-1	Lymphocytes	Tax vmRNA, TAX, vmiRNA	Proinflammatory cytokines, damage to neurons	[86, 132, 133]
HPV	Epithelial cells	vmiRNA	Proliferation, apoptosis	[134]
HAV	Hepatocytes	HAV gRNA, HAV particles	Immune evasion, increased viral infectivity	[31, 117, 135]
HBV	Hepatocytes	vDNA, vRNA, HBsAg	Immune evasion	[118, 136]
HCV	Hepatocytes	HCV gRNA, vmiRNA, vRNA	Immune evasion	[29, 124, 137]
RVFV	WBC	v-protein, vmRNA	Apoptosis, immune evasion	[138]

Viral-infected cells have been shown to shed exosomes containing cellular and viral-specific components. Table lists viral components that have been detected in exosomes. These include viral mRNAs, microRNAs (vmiRNA), non-protein coding RNAs (vRNA), full-length genomic RNA (gRNA), as well as virus-specific proteins. Depending on the exosomal cargo and type of recipient cells, different biological changes may be induced. *Abbreviations*: EBV, Epstein-Barr virus; HSV, herpes simplex virus; CMV, cytomegalovirus; HIV, human immunodeficiency virus; HTLV, human T-lymphotropic virus; HPV, human papillomavirus; HAV, hepatitis A virus; HBV, hepatitis B virus; HCV, hepatitis C virus; RVFV, Rift Valley fever virus.

Table 1. Exosomes, their viral cargo, and their potential role in virus-mediated pathogenesis.

Another virus which has attracted considerable attention is HIV. There are over 38 million people living with HIV, and there is still no cure [74]. Analysis of exosomes released from HIV-1-infected and non-infected cells shows that they differ in their densities [75]. This implies that the contents of the exosomes from infected and non-infected cells are clearly different [60, 61]. Although retroviruses are much smaller than herpesviruses, they are nevertheless

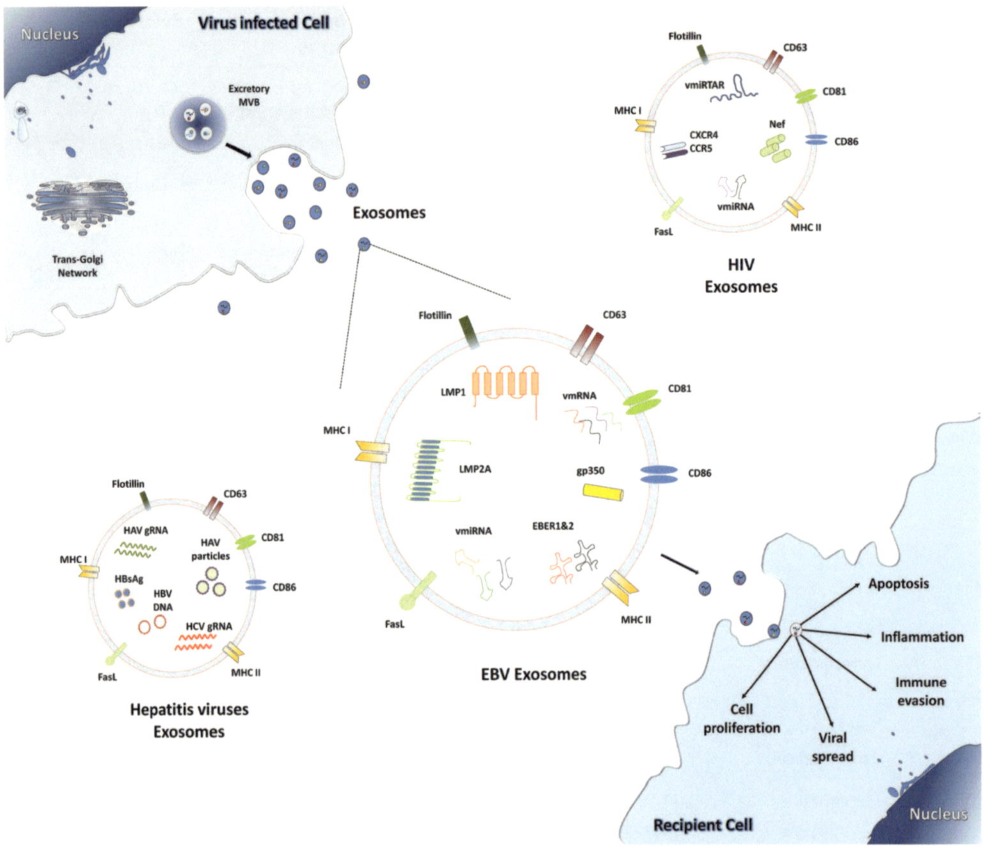

Figure 1. Viruses hijacking the exosomal pathway. Many different viruses have been shown to exploit the exosomal pathway to aid in their infection, spread, and pathogenesis. Three examples are illustrated here. EBV, a dsDNA virus of the herpes family, has been shown to export numerous viral microRNA (vmiRNA), viral mRNA, non-protein coding RNAs (EBERSs), latent membrane proteins (LMP-1 and 2A), and the envelop glycoprotein (gp350). Similarly, other viruses such as HIV, hepatitis A, B and C can also package their proteins and RNAs in exosomes. For HAV and HCV, full-length genomic RNA has been shown to be present in exosomes, which in the case of HCV has been demonstrated to be infectious and capable of producing virus particles.

still slightly larger than exosomes and as such it is unlikely that mature infectious HIV-1 particles could be packaged and excreted within exosomes. However, there is mounting evidence that HIV-1 egress is partly mediated by the endosomal pathway, and both exosomes and HIV-1 are released together in the same fraction [76]. HIV-1 Gag protein has been shown to interact with the exosomal membrane tetraspanins, CD63 and CD81, aiding in the assembly and exit of HIV-1 from infected cells [77–80]. Moreover, several functionally active HIV-1 components have also been shown to be excreted out of infected cells using the exosomal "bus" (**Figure 1**). Once released, exosomes can bind to neighboring cells, travel passively through the blood stream to distant sites, and induce biological changes depending on the nature of the cargo they carry (**Figure 1**) [42]. Nef is one HIV-1 protein that has been shown to be released within exosomes [81]. Studies indicate that Nef plays an important role in activating resting bystander CD4^{+} T cells making them susceptible to HIV infection and viral replication [81–83]. Reports have indicated that HIV-1 may also facilitate its spread to other cells by secreting viral co-receptors, CCR5 and CXCR4, in exosomes [84, 85]. In addition to functional proteins, exosomes from HIV-1-infected cells have been shown to carry several viral miRNAs, including vmiRTAR transcripts, vmiR88 and vmiR99 [23]. Similarly, another human retrovirus, the human T-lymphotropic virus 1 (HTLV-1), also appears to export viral components via the exosomal transport systems. Exosomes released from HTLV-1-infected cells contain not only viral mRNA transcripts, such as those for Tax, HBZ, and Env, but also the biologically active trans-activator protein, Tax [86, 87]. Moreover, HTLV-1 Tax protein has been demonstrated in exosomes isolated from cerebrospinal fluid of patients with HTLV-1-associated myelopathy/tropical spastic paraparesis, suggesting that HTLV-1 may modulate its microenvironment by selective secretion of specific viral cargo [88].

The list of components of cellular and microbial origin detected in exosomes is constantly expanding. This has led to the establishment of several online databases to catalogue the contents of exosomes. There is now substantial evidence indicating that many different types of pathogens, including bacteria, viruses, parasites, and even prions, can exploit the exosomal pathway [89, 90]. Of the viruses, members belonging to families as diverse as *Bunyaviridae* (enveloped RNA viruses) and *Papillomaviridae* (non-enveloped DNA viruses) have been shown to export their products in exosomes (**Table 1**). Moreover, studies are beginning to address the functional impact of exosomes carrying viral cargo in the pathogenesis of viral infections. One major challenge is to understand the mechanisms that regulate the selection of cargo to be packaged into exosomes and how we can use exosomes as biomarkers for viral infections and disease progression [89, 91].

3. Role of exosomes in viral pathogenesis

Exosomes released by viral-infected cells contain not only viral components, but also those of cellular origin [23, 67, 89]. It appears that viruses are able not only to export their own products in exosomes, but also to somehow influence which cellular products are packaged within the excretory vesicles. This is evident by the findings that exosomal cargo of cellular origin is clearly different from non-infected cells of the same type [60, 61, 92]. Thus, any pathophysiological impact of viral exosomes on recipient cells is by no means due to viral components only. An accumulating body of data indicates that exosomes from viral-infected cells can induce processes as diverse as immune evasion, apoptosis, proliferation, transcellular spread, and cytokine modulation (**Table 1**). The molecular details of how these processes are triggered are poorly understood and most probably dependent on multiple factors, including the type of cells releasing/receiving exosomes, nature of the exosomal cargo, mode of delivery, and stage of infection [1, 90]. This probably explains why apparently contradicting results have been reported in different studies [93, 94]. For EBV, it has been shown that uninfected epithelial cells exposed to exosomes derived from infected B cells are internalized via caveolar-dependent endocytosis and induce physiological changes in these cells [95]. Studies reported that exosomes derived from nasopharyngeal carcinoma (NPC) and from EBV-immortalized lymphoblastoid cell lines (LCLs) either inhibit proliferation of EBV-reactive CD4+ cells or induce apoptosis [70, 93, 96]. Similar results were observed with exosomes isolated from EBV-associated NPC patients and mice xenografted with NPC [97]. These pathophysiological changes were suggested to be due to viral and cellular components such as LMP-1, LMP-2A, viral miRNAs, and cellular galectin 9, excreted in exosomes from EBV-infected cells [72, 93, 97, 98]. The finding of EBV LMP-1 in exosomes is noteworthy [70, 93]. This is a well-known oncoprotein that plays a key role in the immortalization of EBV-infected cells [99]. Not surprisingly, LMP-1 has been extensively studied and shown to function as a constitutively activated receptor, signaling through the TRAF pathway leading to the activation of the master transcription factor, NFκB [100, 101]. LMP-2A is also an EBV latent protein expressed on the plasma membrane of latently infected cells [102]. Like LMP-1, LMP-2A also appears to be a constitutively activated receptor; while LMP-1 mimics CD40 receptor, LMP-2A mimics activated B-cell receptor (BCR), allowing infected cells to develop and survive, even in the absence of BCR signaling [103, 104]. Although it is not known how these membrane proteins are selected for export in exosomes, or what their functional impact is on recipient cells, it is tempting to postulate that the cell survival signals provided by LMP-2A and cell proliferation signals provided by LMP-1, if transferable to recipient cells, would be important in EBV pathogenesis.

Recently, we reported that exosomes from both EBV-infected and non-infected B cells are taken up by recipient cells, but only the exosomes from EBV-infected cells induced apoptosis in recipient cells in a dose-dependent manner [92]. We further showed that apoptosis was induced via the activation of the extrinsic pathway involving Fas-ligand (Fas-L) present in EBV exosomes. Moreover, the process could be blocked by using anti-Fas-L antibodies [92]. Another study reported that LCL-derived exosomes contain Fas-L and MHCII molecules and induce apoptosis in autologous CD4+ T cells [96]. Taken together, these studies indicate that one mechanism by which EBV could evade the body's immune system may be by shedding exosomes containing signals that inhibit proliferation and/or promote apoptosis of anti–EBV-infiltrating lymphocytes. The fact that similar effects on bystander cells, albeit through different mechanisms, have also been reported for exosomes released from rotavirus and HIV-1–infected cells [105, 106] supports this hypothesis.

Another well-known mechanism by which some viruses can evade the immune responses is by down-regulating the expression of viral lytic genes and persisting in the infected cells in a latent state [107]. It's a simple strategy; no viral antigens expressed in infected cells means no immune system can be triggered [108]. In this context, herpesviruses are among the most extensively studied [109, 110]. For example, herpes simplex type 1 (HSV-1) replicates in mucosal epithelial cells during primary infection and then enters sensory neurons where it establishes life-long latency [111]. During the latent state, although no viral proteins are expressed, numerous vmiRNAs have been detected, and some of these vmiRNAs appear to be central in suppressing viral gene expression and maintaining latency [112–114]. The complexity of this process has been further exposed by recent findings indicating that HSV-1 can excrete vmiRNAs in exosomes, which on transfer to recipient cells, can suppress viral gene expression and viral spread to uninfected cells [115]. Furthermore, HSV-1 can also transfer antiviral factors, such as STING (stimulator of IFN genes), to suppress its cell-to-cell spread in circumstances that may be unfavorable [116]. Thus, inhibiting viral replication and spread in the face of a competent immune threat could be an important strategy for viruses to escape immune elimination and persist.

In some viral infections, such as with hepatitis B (HBV), non-infectious subviral particles are released into the serum, often at levels 1000s of fold higher compared to mature infectious particles [117, 118]. In evolutionary terms, it does not make sense why a virus would opt to shed enormous amounts of non-infectious subviral particles if it was not beneficial for the virus. One plausible hypothesis is that such subviral particles act as a decoy to divert the immune responses away from the bonafide infectious virions [118, 119]. HSV-1-infected cells can also release subviral particles, referred to as the L-particles. These particles have neither viral capsid nor viral DNA, and they are not infectious, but they do contain several HSV proteins [120, 121]. Recent studies suggest that the transfer of L particles to bystander cells can modulate the microenvironment to facilitate immune evasion and viral infection [122]. Similarly, there is evidence that some viruses can manipulate their microenvironment by secreting exosomes containing cargo that interferes with the host inflammatory and antiviral factors [119, 123].

In addition to immune modulation, exosomes released from some viral-infected cells can promote infection and enhance viral spread. A good example of this is HIV-1. Exosome-mediated transfer of HIV-1 co-receptors CCR5 and CXCR4 to recipient cells that do not normally express these receptors can facilitate HIV-1 infection in these cells [84, 85]. In the case of hepatitis C virus, it has been reported that infected cells release exosomes containing full-length viral genomic RNA as well as viral-specific proteins [29, 30, 124]. Importantly, HCV RNA carrying exosomes could transmit the infection to non-infected cells and establish a productive infection [29, 30, 124]. This receptor-independent mechanism of HCV transmission would prevent the virus from being exposed to antibodies that would normally be effective in neutralizing cell-free virus [125, 126]. Some viruses can also manipulate with the endocytic pathway, not for export of their cargo, but for virion assembly and egress from the infected cells during replication. For example, HSV-1 can interact with Rab27a via its tegument protein and its glycoproteins gH and gD [55]. Depletion of Rab27a results in significant reduction in both viral production and viral egress, highlighting the importance of the Rab27a in the egress of HSV-1 [55]. A similar phenomenon has been reported for several other members of the *herpesviridae* family, including cytomegalovirus (CMV) and human herpesvirus 6 (HHV-6) [23].

Although we have focused on how viruses exploit the exosome system to aid their infection and pathogenesis, it should be borne in mind that the shedding of exosomes is a normal physiological process and it also plays a role in defending against infections [90, 127]. For example, a recent study reported that exosomes isolated from semen, but not from blood of healthy individuals, were able to inhibit the replication of HIV-1 in *in vitro* culture [42]. Remarkably, this anti-viral activity of semen exosomes appeared to be restricted to retroviruses and had no effect on HSV-1 or HSV-2 replication [5]. Ironically, some viruses are able to not only overcome these defense mechanisms but also exploit them to their benefit.

4. Conclusions

Our current understanding of microvesicle biology and function, especially in regard to virus infections, is still in its early stages. The study of viral exosomes has shown that the transfer of viral and cellular factors in exosomes enables the manipulation of the neighboring unaffected cells. Microvesicle-mediated communication allows the virus to respond and control the cellular microenvironment. A number of reports suggest that viruses utilize the cellular vesiculation pathway for virus budding/assembly, immune evasion, and intercellular communication. Understanding the role of exosomes in the host-viral interactions can open new avenues of understanding the disease mechanisms and future diagnostic and therapeutic interventions.

Acknowledgements

The work in Khan Laboratory is supported by grants 31R90, 31016, and 31M263 from UAEU.

Author details

Gulfaraz Khan*, Waqar Ahmed and Pretty S. Philip

*Address all correspondence to: g_khan@uaeu.ac.ae

Department of Microbiology and Immunology, College of Medicine and Health Sciences, United Arab Emirates University, Al Ain, United Arab Emirates

References

[1] van der Pol E, Böing AN, Harrison P, Sturk A, Nieuwland R. Classification, functions, and clinical relevance of extracellular vesicles. Pharmacological Reviews. 2012;**64**:676-705

[2] De Toro J, Herschlik L, Waldner C, Mongini C. Emerging roles of exosomes in normal and pathological conditions: New insights for diagnosis and therapeutic applications. Frontiers in Immunology. 2015;**6**:203

[3] Lässer C, Seyed Alikhani V, Ekström K, Eldh M, Torregrosa Paredes P, Bossios A, Sjöstrand M, Gabrielsson S, Lötvall J, Valadi H. Human saliva, plasma and breast milk exosomes contain RNA: Uptake by macrophages. Journal of Translational Medicine. 2011;**9**:9

[4] Street JM, Barran PE, Mackay CL, Weidt S, Balmforth C, Walsh TS, Chalmers RT, Webb DJ, Dear JW. Identification and proteomic profiling of exosomes in human cerebrospinal fluid. Journal of Translational Medicine. 2012;**10**:5

[5] Madison MN, Roller RJ, Okeoma CM. Human semen contains exosomes with potent anti-HIV-1 activity. Retrovirology. 2014;**11**:102

[6] Villanueva MT. Microenvironment: Small containers, important cargo. Nature Reviews Cancer. 2014;**14**:764

[7] Pant S, Hilton H, Burczynski ME. The multifaceted exosome: Biogenesis, role in normal and aberrant cellular function, and frontiers for pharmacological and biomarker opportunities. Biochemical Pharmacology. 2012;**83**:1484-1494

[8] Robbins PD, Morelli AE. Regulation of immune responses by extracellular vesicles. Nature Reviews Immunology. 2014;**14**:195-208

[9] Hurley JH, Odorizzi G. Get on the exosome bus with ALIX. Nature Cell Biology. 2012;**14**: 654-655

[10] Stoorvogel W. Resolving sorting mechanisms into exosomes. Cell Research. 2015;**25**(5): 531-532

[11] Raiborg C, Stenmark H. The ESCRT machinery in endosomal sorting of ubiquitylated membrane proteins. Nature. 2009;**458**:445-452

[12] Hurley JH. The ESCRT complexes. Critical Reviews in Biochemistry and Molecular Biology. 2010;**45**:463-487

[13] Colombo M, Raposo G, Théry C. Biogenesis, secretion, and intercellular interactions of exosomes and other extracellular vesicles. Annual Review of Cell and Developmental Biology. 2014;**30**:255-289

[14] Votteler J, Sundquist WI. Virus budding and the ESCRT pathway. Cell Host & Microbe. 2013;**14**:232-241

[15] van Niel G, Charrin S, Simoes S, Romao M, Rochin L, Saftig P, Marks MS, Rubinstein E, Raposo G. The tetraspanin CD63 regulates ESCRT-independent and -dependent endosomal sorting during melanogenesis. Developmental Cell. 2011;**21**:708-721

[16] Trajkovic K, Hsu C, Chiantia S, Rajendran L, Wenzel D, Wieland F, Schwille P, Brügger B, Simons M. Ceramide triggers budding of exosome vesicles into multivesicular endosomes. Science. 2008;**319**:1244-1247

[17] Ghossoub R, Lembo F, Rubio A, Gaillard CB, Bouchet J, Vitale N, Slavík J, Machala M, Zimmermann P. Syntenin-ALIX exosome biogenesis and budding into multivesicular bodies are controlled by ARF6 and PLD2. Nature Communications. 2014;**5**:3477

[18] Chavrier P, Parton RG, Hauri HP, Simons K, Zerial M. Localization of low molecular weight GTP binding proteins to exocytic and endocytic compartments. Cell. 1990;**62**: 317-329

[19] Vitelli R, Santillo M, Lattero D, Chiariello M, Bifulco M, Bruni CB, Bucci C. Role of the small GTPase Rab7 in the late endocytic pathway. Journal of Biological Chemistry. 1997;**272**:4391-4397

[20] Zerial M, McBride H. Rab proteins as membrane organizers. Nature Reviews Molecular Cell Biology. 2001;**2**:107-117

[21] Gruenberg J. Viruses and endosome membrane dynamics. Current Opinion in Cell Biology. 2009;**21**:582-588

[22] de Armas-Rillo L, Valera M-S, Marrero-Hernández S, Valenzuela-Fernández A. Membrane dynamics associated with viral infection. Reviews in Medical Virology. 2016;**26**:146-160

[23] Alenquer M, Amorim MJ. Exosome biogenesis, regulation, and function in viral infection. Viruses. 2015;**7**:5066-5083

[24] Nour AM, Modis Y. Endosomal vesicles as vehicles for viral genomes. Trends in Cell Biology. 2014;**24**:449-454

[25] Piccini LE, Castilla V, Damonte EB. Dengue-3 virus entry into vero cells: Role of clathrin-mediated endocytosis in the outcome of infection. PloS One. 2015;**10**:e0140824

[26] Smit JM, Moesker B, Rodenhuis-Zybert I, Wilschut J. Flavivirus cell Entry and membrane fusion. Viruses. 2011;**3**:160-171

[27] Hamel R, Dejarnac O, Wichit S, Ekchariyawat P, Neyret A, Luplertlop N, Perera-Lecoin M, Surasombatpattana P, Talignani L, Thomas F, Cao-Lormeau V-M, Choumet V, Briant L, Desprès P, Amara A, Yssel H, Missé D. Biology of zika virus infection in human skin cells. Journal of Virology. 2015;**89**:8880-8896

[28] Cohen FS. How viruses invade cells. Biophysical Journal. 2016;**110**:1028-1032

[29] Ramakrishnaiah V, Thumann C, Fofana I, Habersetzer F, Pan Q, Ruiter PE de, Willemsen R, Demmers JAA, Raj VS, Jenster G, Kwekkeboom J, Tilanus HW, Haagmans BL, Baumert TF, Laan LJW van der. Exosome-mediated transmission of hepatitis C virus between human hepatoma Huh7.5 cells. Proceedings of the National Academy of Sciences 2013;**110**:13109-13113

[30] Longatti A, Boyd B, Chisari FV. Virion-independent transfer of replication-competent hepatitis C virus RNA between permissive cells. Journal of Virology. 2015;**89**:2956-2961

[31] Longatti A. The dual role of exosomes in hepatitis A and C virus transmission and viral immune activation. Viruses. 2015;**7**:6707-6715

[32] Izquierdo-Useros N, Naranjo-Gomez M, Erkizia I, Puertas MC, Borras FE, Blanco J, Martinez-Picado J. HIV and mature dendritic cells: Trojan exosomes riding the trojan horse? PLOS Pathogens 2010;**6**(3):e1000740

[33] Gould SJ, Booth AM, Hildreth JEK. The Trojan exosome hypothesis. Proceedings of the National Academy of Sciences. 2003;**100**:10592-10597

[34] Wiley RD, Gummuluru S. Immature dendritic cell-derived exosomes can mediate HIV-1 trans infection. Proceedings of the National Academy of Sciences of the United States of America. 2006;**103**:738-743

[35] Piguet V, Steinman RM. The interaction of HIV with dendritic cells: Outcomes and pathways. Trends in Immunology. 2007;**28**:503-510

[36] Welsch S, Keppler OT, Habermann A, Allespach I, Krijnse-Locker J, Kräusslich H-G. HIV-1 buds predominantly at the plasma membrane of primary human macrophages. PLOS Pathogens. 2007;**3**:e36

[37] Woodward CL, Cheng SN, Jensen GJ. Electron cryo-tomography studies of maturing HIV-1 particles reveal the assembly pathway of the viral core. Journal of Virology. 2014:JVI.02997-14

[38] Yandrapalli N, Muriaux D, Favard C. Lipid domains in HIV-1 assembly. Frontiers in Microbiology. 2014;**5**:220

[39] Chahar HS, Bao X, Casola A. Exosomes and their role in the life cycle and pathogenesis of RNA viruses. Viruses. 2015;**7**:3204-3225

[40] Anderson MR, Kashanchi F, Jacobson S. Exosomes in viral disease. Neurotherapeutics. 2016;**13**:535-546

[41] Meng B, Ip NCY, Prestwood LJ, Abbink TEM, Lever AML. Evidence that the endosomal sorting complex required for transport-II (ESCRT-II) is required for efficient human immunodeficiency virus-1 (HIV-1) production. Retrovirology. 2015;**12**:72

[42] Madison MN, Okeoma CM. Exosomes: Implications in HIV-1 pathogenesis. Viruses. 2015;**7**:4093-4118

[43] Mori Y, Koike M, Moriishi E, Kawabata A, Tang H, Oyaizu H, Uchiyama Y, Yamanishi K. Human herpesvirus-6 induces MVB formation, and virus egress occurs by an exosomal release pathway. Traffic 2008;**9**:1728-1742

[44] Savina A, Vidal M, Colombo MI. The exosome pathway in K562 cells is regulated by Rab11. Journal of Cell Science. 2002;**115**(Pt 12):2505-2515

[45] Bruce EA, Digard P, Stuart AD. The Rab11 pathway is required for influenza A virus budding and filament formation. Journal of Virology. 2010;**84**:5848-5859

[46] Rowe RK, Suszko JW, Pekosz A. Roles for the recycling endosome, Rab8, and Rab11 in hantavirus release from epithelial cells. Virology. 2008;**382**:239-249

[47] Utley TJ, Ducharme NA, Varthakavi V, Shepherd BE, Santangelo PJ, Lindquist ME, Goldenring JR, Crowe JE. Respiratory syncytial virus uses a Vps4-independent budding mechanism controlled by Rab11-FIP2. Proceedings of the National Academy of Sciences of the United States of America. 2008;**105**:10209-10214

[48] Abrami L, Brandi L, Moayeri M, Brown MJ, Krantz BA, Leppla SH, Goot FG. Hijacking multivesicular bodies enables long-term and exosome-mediated long-distance action of anthrax toxin. Cell Reports. 2013;**5**:986-996

[49] Bhuin T, Roy JK. Rab11 in disease progression. International Journal of Molecular and Cellular Medicine. 2015;**4**:1-8

[50] Ostrowski M, Carmo NB, Krumeich S, Fanget I, Raposo G, Savina A, Moita CF, Schauer K, Hume AN, Freitas RP, Goud B, Benaroch P, Hacohen N, Fukuda M, Desnos C, Seabra MC, Darchen F, Amigorena S, Moita LF, Thery C. Rab27a and Rab27b control different steps of the exosome secretion pathway. Nature Cell Biology. 2010;**12**:19-30

[51] Bobrie A, Krumeich S, Reyal F, Recchi C, Moita LF, Seabra MC, Ostrowski M, Théry C. Rab27a supports exosome-dependent and -independent mechanisms that modify the tumor microenvironment and can promote tumor progression. Cancer Research. 2012;**72**:4920-4930

[52] Fraile-Ramos A, Cepeda V, Elstak E, Sluijs P. Rab27a is required for human cytomegalovirus assembly. PloS One. 2010;**5**:e15318

[53] Gerber PP, Cabrini M, Jancic C, Paoletti L, Banchio C, Bilderling C, Sigaut L, Pietrasanta LI, Duette G, Freed EO, Basile G de S, Moita CF, Moita LF, Amigorena S, Benaroch P, Geffner J, Ostrowski M. Rab27a controls HIV-1 assembly by regulating plasma membrane levels of phosphatidylinositol 4,5-bisphosphate. Journal of Cell Biology. 2015;**209**:435-452

[54] Miranda-Saksena M, Boadle RA, Aggarwal A, Tijono B, Rixon FJ, Diefenbach RJ, Cunningham AL. Herpes simplex virus utilizes the large secretory vesicle pathway for anterograde transport of tegument and envelope proteins and for viral exocytosis from growth cones of human fetal axons. Journal of Virology. 2009;**83**:3187-3199

[55] Bello-Morales R, Crespillo AJ, Fraile-Ramos A, Tabarés E, Alcina A, López-Guerrero JA. Role of the small GTPase Rab27a during herpes simplex virus infection of oligodendrocytic cells. BMC Microbiology 2012;**12**:265

[56] White IJ, Bailey LM, Aghakhani MR, Moss SE, Futter CE. EGF stimulates annexin 1-dependent inward vesiculation in a multivesicular endosome subpopulation. The EMBO Journal. 2006;**25**:1-12

[57] Morales-Sánchez A, Fuentes-Pananá EM. Human viruses and cancer. Viruses. 2014;**6**: 4047-4079

[58] Chugh PE, Sin S-H, Ozgur S, Henry DH, Menezes P, Griffith J, Eron JJ, Damania B, Dittmer DP. Systemically circulating viral and tumor-derived microRNAs in KSHV-associated malignancies. PLOS Pathogens. 2013;**9**:e1003484

[59] Canitano A, Venturi G, Borghi M, Ammendolia MG, Fais S. Exosomes released in vitro from Epstein–Barr virus (EBV)-infected cells contain EBV-encoded latent phase mRNAs. Cancer Letters. 2013;**337**:193-199

[60] Meckes Jr DG, Gunawardena HP, Dekroon RM, Heaton PR, Edwards RH, Ozgur S, Griffith JD, Damania B, Raab-Traub N. Modulation of B-cell exosome proteins by gamma herpesvirus infection. Proceedings of the National Academy of Sciences of the United States of America. 2013;**110**:E2925-2933

[61] Hoshina S, Sekizuka T, Kataoka M, Hasegawa H, Hamada H, Kuroda M, Katano H. Profile of exosomal and intracellular microRNA in gamma-herpesvirus-infected lymphoma cell lines. PLOS ONE 2016;**11**:e0162574

[62] Pfeffer S, Zavolan M, Grässer FA, Chien M, Russo JJ, Ju J, John B, Enright AJ, Marks D, Sander C, Tuschl T. Identification of virus-encoded microRNAs. Science 2004;**304**:734-736

[63] Pegtel DM, Cosmopoulos K, Thorley-Lawson DA, Eijndhoven MAJ van, Hopmans ES, Lindenberg JL, Gruijl TD de, Würdinger T, Middeldorp JM. Functional delivery of viral miRNAs via exosomes. Proceedings of the National Academy of Sciences. 2010;**107**:6328-6333

[64] Edwards RH, Marquitz AR, Raab-Traub N. Epstein-Barr virus BART microRNAs are produced from a large intron prior to splicing. Journal of Virology. 2008;**82**:9094-9106

[65] Hooykaas MJG, Kruse E, Wiertz EJHJ, Lebbink RJ. Comprehensive profiling of functional Epstein-Barr virus miRNA expression in human cell lines. BMC Genomics. 2016;**17**:644

[66] Shinozaki-Ushiku A, Kunita A, Isogai M, Hibiya T, Ushiku T, Takada K, Fukayama M. Profiling of virus-encoded microRNAs in Epstein-Barr virus-associated gastric carcinoma and their roles in gastric carcinogenesis. Journal of Virology. 2015;**89**:5581-5591

[67] Gallo A, Vella S, Miele M, Timoneri F, Di Bella M, Bosi S, Sciveres M, Conaldi PG. Global profiling of viral and cellular non-coding RNAs in Epstein-Barr virus-induced lymphoblastoid cell lines and released exosome cargos. Cancer Letters. 2017;**388**:334-343

[68] Ahmed W, Philip PS, Tariq S, Khan G. Epstein-Barr virus-encoded small RNAs (EBERs) are present in fractions related to exosomes released by EBV-transformed cells. PloS One. 2014;**9**:e99163

[69] Iwakiri D, Zhou L, Samanta M, Matsumoto M, Ebihara T, Seya T, Imai S, Fujieda M, Kawa K, Takada K. Epstein-Barr virus (EBV)-encoded small RNA is released from EBV-infected cells and activates signaling from toll-like receptor 3. Journal of Experimental Medicine. 2009;**206**(10):2091-2099

[70] Flanagan J, Middeldorp J, Sculley T. Localization of the Epstein-Barr virus protein LMP 1 to exosomes. Journal of General Virology. 2003;**84**(Pt 7):1871-1879

[71] Verweij FJ, van Eijndhoven MAJ, Hopmans ES, Vendrig T, Wurdinger T, Cahir-McFarland E, Kieff E, Geerts D, van der Kant R, Neefjes J, Middeldorp JM, Pegtel DM. LMP1 association with CD63 in endosomes and secretion via exosomes limits constitutive NF-κB activation. The EMBO Journal. 2011;**30**:2115-2129

[72] Ikeda M, Longnecker R. Cholesterol is critical for Epstein-Barr virus latent membrane protein 2A trafficking and protein stability. Virology. 2007;**360**:461-468

[73] Vallhov H, Gutzeit C, Johansson SM, Nagy N, Paul M, Li Q, Friend S, George TC, Klein E, Scheynius A, Gabrielsson S. Exosomes containing glycoprotein 350 released by EBV-transformed B cells selectively target B cells through CD21 and block EBV infection in vitro. Journal of Immunology. 2011;**186**:73-82

[74] GBD 2015 HIV Collaborators, Wang H, Wolock TM, Carter A, Nguyen G, Kyu HH, Gakidou E, Hay SI, Mills EJ, Trickey A, Msemburi W, Coates MM, Mooney MD, Fraser MS, Sligar A, Salomon J, Larson HJ, Friedman J, Abajobir AA, Abate KH, Abbas KM, Razek MMAE, Abd-Allah F, Abdulle AM, Abera SF, Abubakar I, Abu-Raddad LJ, Abu-Rmeileh NME, Abyu GY, Adebiyi AO, et al. Estimates of global, regional, and national incidence, prevalence, and mortality of HIV, 1980-2015: the Global Burden of Disease Study 2015. The Lancet HIV. 2016;**3**:e361-387

[75] Cantin R, Diou J, Bélanger D, Tremblay AM, Gilbert C. Discrimination between exosomes and HIV-1: Purification of both vesicles from cell-free supernatants. Journal of Immunological Methods 2008;**338**:21-30

[76] Wu L, KewalRamani VN. Dendritic-cell interactions with HIV: Infection and viral dissemination. Nature Reviews Immunology. 2006;**6**:859-868

[77] Grigorov B, Attuil-Audenis V, Perugi F, Nedelec M, Watson S, Pique C, Darlix J-L, Conjeaud H, Muriaux D. A role for CD81 on the late steps of HIV-1 replication in a chronically infected T cell line. Retrovirology. 2009;**6**:28

[78] Izquierdo-Useros N, Naranjo-Gómez M, Archer J, Hatch SC, Erkizia I, Blanco J, Borràs FE, Puertas MC, Connor JH, Fernández-Figueras MT, Moore L, Clotet B, Gummuluru S, Martinez-Picado J. Capture and transfer of HIV-1 particles by mature dendritic cells converges with the exosome-dissemination pathway. Blood. 2009;**113**:2732-2741

[79] Jolly C, Sattentau QJ. Human immunodeficiency virus type 1 assembly, budding, and cell-cell spread in T cells take place in tetraspanin-enriched plasma membrane domains. Journal of Virology. 2007;**81**:7873-7884

[80] Sato K, Aoki J, Misawa N, Daikoku E, Sano K, Tanaka Y, Koyanagi Y. Modulation of human immunodeficiency virus type 1 infectivity through incorporation of tetraspanin proteins. Journal of Virology. 2008;**82**:1021-1033

[81] Campbell TD, Khan M, Huang M-B, Bond VC, Powell MD. HIV-1 Nef protein is secreted into vesicles that can fuse with target cells and virions. Ethnicity & Disease. 2008;**18**(2 Suppl 2):S2-14-19

[82] Carvalho JV, Castro RO, Silva EZM, Silveira PP, Silva-Januário ME, Arruda E, Jamur MC, Oliver C, Aguiar RS, daSilva LLP. Nef neutralizes the ability of exosomes from CD4+ T cells to act as decoys during HIV-1 infection. PloS One. 2014;**9**:e113691

[83] Arenaccio C, Chiozzini C, Columba-Cabezas S, Manfredi F, Affabris E, Baur A, Federico M. Exosomes from human immunodeficiency virus type 1 (HIV-1)-infected cells license quiescent CD4+ T lymphocytes To replicate HIV-1 through a Nef- and ADAM17-dependent mechanism. Journal of Virology. 2014;**88**:11529-11539

[84] Mack M, Kleinschmidt A, Brühl H, Klier C, Nelson PJ, Cihak J, Plachý J, Stangassinger M, Erfle V, Schlöndorff D. Transfer of the chemokine receptor CCR5 between cells by membrane-derived microparticles: A mechanism for cellular human immunodeficiency virus 1 infection. Nature Medicine. 2000;**6**:769-775

[85] Rozmyslowicz T, Majka M, Kijowski J, Murphy SL, Conover DO, Poncz M, Ratajczak J, Gaulton GN, Ratajczak MZ. Platelet- and megakaryocyte-derived microparticles transfer CXCR4 receptor to CXCR4-null cells and make them susceptible to infection by X4-HIV. AIDS (London, England). 2003;**17**:33-42

[86] Jaworski E, Narayanan A, Van Duyne R, Shabbeer-Meyering S, Iordanskiy S, Saifuddin M, Das R, Afonso PV, Sampey GC, Chung M, Popratiloff A, Shrestha B, Sehgal M, Jain P, Vertes A, Mahieux R, Kashanchi F. Human T-lymphotropic virus type 1-infected cells secrete exosomes that contain Tax protein. Journal of Biological Chemistry. 2014;**289**: 22284-22305

[87] Narayanan A, Jaworski E, Van Duyne R, Iordanskiy S, Guendel I, Das R, Currer R, Sampey G, Chung M, Kehn-Hall K, Bailey C, Popratiloff A, Kashanchi F. Exosomes derived from HTLV-1 infected cells contain the viral protein Tax. Retrovirology. 2014;**11**(Suppl 1):O46

[88] Anderson M, Lepene B, Kashanchi F, Jacobson S. Detection of human T-cell lymphotropic virus type I proteins in exosomes from HAM/TSP patient CSF by novel nanotrap technology (I7-5E). Neurology 2015;**84**(14 Supplement):I7-5E

[89] Fleming A, Sampey G, Chung M-C, Bailey C, van Hoek ML, Kashanchi F, Hakami RM. The carrying pigeons of the cell: Exosomes and their role in infectious diseases caused by human pathogens. Pathogens and Disease. 2014;**71**:109-120

[90] Schorey JS, Cheng Y, Singh PP, Smith VL. Exosomes and other extracellular vesicles in host–pathogen interactions. EMBO Reports. 2015;**16**:24-43

[91] Soung YH, Ford S, Zhang V, Chung J. Exosomes in cancer diagnostics. Cancers. 2017;**9**(1): pii:E8

[92] Ahmed W, Philip PS, Attoub S, Khan G. Epstein-Barr virus infected cells release Fas-ligand in exosomal fractions and induce apoptosis in recipient cells via the extrinsic pathway. Journal of General Virology. 2015;**96**:3646-3659

[93] Keryer-Bibens C, Pioche-Durieu C, Villemant C, Souquere S, Nishi N, Hirashima M, Middeldorp J, Busson P. Exosomes released by EBV-infected nasopharyngeal carcinoma cells convey the viral Latent Membrane Protein 1 and the immunomodulatory protein galectin 9. BMC Cancer. 2006;**6**:283

[94] Gutzeit C, Nagy N, Gentile M, Lyberg K, Gumz J, Vallhov H, Puga I, Klein E, Gabrielsson S, Cerutti A, Scheynius A. Exosomes derived from Burkitt's lymphoma cell lines induce proliferation, differentiation, and class-switch recombination in B Cells. Journal of Immunology. 2014;**192**:5852-5862

[95] Nanbo A, Kawanishi E, Yoshida R, Yoshiyama H. Exosomes derived from Epstein-Barr virus-infected cells are internalized via caveola-dependent endocytosis and promote phenotypic modulation in target cells. Journal of Virology. 2013;**87**:10334-10347

[96] Klinker MW, Lizzio V, Reed TJ, Fox DA, Lundy SK. Human B cell-derived lymphoblastoid cell lines constitutively produce fas ligand and secrete MHCII+FasL+ Killer exosomes. Frontiers in Immunology. 2014;**5**:1-10

[97] Klibi J, Niki T, Riedel A, Pioche-Durieu C, Souquere S, Rubinstein E, Le Moulec S, Moulec SLE, Guigay J, Hirashima M, Guemira F, Adhikary D, Mautner J, Busson P. Blood diffusion and Th1-suppressive effects of galectin-9-containing exosomes released by Epstein-Barr virus-infected nasopharyngeal carcinoma cells. Blood. 2009;**113**:1957-1966

[98] Meckes DG. Exosomal communication goes viral. Journal of Virology. 2015;**89**:5200-5203

[99] Wang D, Liebowitz D, Kieff E. An EBV membrane protein expressed in immortalized lymphocytes transforms established rodent cells. Cell. 1985;**43**(3 Pt 2):831-840

[100] Mosialos G, Birkenbach M, Yalamanchili R, VanArsdale T, Ware C, Kieff E. The Epstein-Barr virus transforming protein LMP1 engages signaling proteins for the tumor necrosis factor receptor family. Cell. 1995;**80**:389-399

[101] Lavorgna A, Harhaj EW. EBV LMP1: New and shared pathways to NF-κB activation. Proceedings of the National Academy of Sciences of the United States of America. 2012;**109**:2188-2189

[102] Longnecker R, Kieff E. A second Epstein-Barr virus membrane protein (LMP2) is expressed in latent infection and colocalizes with LMP1. Journal of Virology. 1990;**64**: 2319-2326

[103] Caldwell RG, Wilson JB, Anderson SJ, Longnecker R. Epstein-Barr virus LMP2A drives B cell development and survival in the absence of normal B cell receptor signals. Immunity. 1998;**9**:405-411

[104] Casola S, Otipoby KL, Alimzhanov M, Humme S, Uyttersprot N, Kutok JL, Carroll MC, Rajewsky K. B cell receptor signal strength determines B cell fate. Nature Immunology. 2004;**5**:317-327

[105] Barreto A, Rodríguez L-S, Rojas OL, Wolf M, Greenberg HB, Franco MA, Angel J. Membrane vesicles released by intestinal epithelial cells infected with rotavirus inhibit T-cell function. Viral Immunology. 2010;**23**:595-608

[106] Lenassi M, Cagney G, Liao M, Vaupotič T, Bartholomeeusen K, Cheng Y, Krogan NJ, Plemenitaš A, Peterlin BM. HIV Nef is secreted in exosomes and triggers apoptosis in bystander CD4+ T cells. Traffic. 2010;**11**:110-122

[107] Oldstone MBA. Viral persistence: Parameters, mechanisms and future predictions. Virology. 2006;**344**:111-118

[108] Cox JE, Sullivan CS. Balance and stealth: The role of noncoding RNAs in the regulation of virus gene expression. Annual Review of Virology. 2014;**1**:89-109

[109] Stern-Ginossar N, Elefant N, Zimmermann A, Wolf DG, Saleh N, Biton M, Horwitz E, Prokocimer Z, Prichard M, Hahn G, Goldman-Wohl D, Greenfield C, Yagel S, Hengel H, Altuvia Y, Margalit H, Mandelboim O. Host immune system gene targeting by a viral miRNA. Science. 2007;**317**:376-381

[110] Cullen BR. MicroRNAs as mediators of viral evasion of the immune system. Nature Immunology. 2013;**14**:205-210

[111] Nicoll MP, Proença JT, Efstathiou S. The molecular basis of herpes simplex virus latency. FEMS Microbiology Reviews. 2012;**36**:684-705

[112] Umbach JL, Kramer MF, Jurak I, Karnowski HW, Coen DM, Cullen BR. MicroRNAs expressed by herpes simplex virus 1 during latent infection regulate viral mRNAs. Nature. 2008;**454**:780-783

[113] Du T, Han Z, Zhou G, Roizman B. Patterns of accumulation of miRNAs encoded by herpes simplex virus during productive infection, latency, and on reactivation. Proceedings of the National Academy of Sciences of the United States of America. 2015;**112**:E49–E55

[114] Piedade D, Azevedo-Pereira JM. The role of microRNAs in the pathogenesis of herpesvirus infection. Viruses. 2016;**8**(6):pii: E156

[115] Han Z, Liu X, Chen X, Zhou X, Du T, Roizman B, Zhou G. miR-H28 and miR-H29 expressed late in productive infection are exported and restrict HSV-1 replication and spread in recipient cells. Proceedings of the National Academy of Sciences of the United States of America. 2016;**113**:E894–E901

[116] Kalamvoki M, Du T, Roizman B. Cells infected with herpes simplex virus 1 export to uninfected cells exosomes containing STING, viral mRNAs, and microRNAs. Proceedings of the National Academy of Sciences of the United States of America. 2014;**111**:E4991-4996

[117] Chai N, Chang HE, Nicolas E, Han Z, Jarnik M, Taylor J. Properties of subviral particles of hepatitis B virus. Journal of Virology. 2008;**82**:7812-7817

[118] Jiang B, Himmelsbach K, Ren H, Boller K, Hildt E. Subviral hepatitis B virus filaments, like infectious viral particles, are released via multivesicular bodies. Journal of Virology. 2016;**90**:3330-3341

[119] Kouwaki T, Fukushima Y, Daito T, Sanada T, Yamamoto N, Mifsud EJ, Leong CR, Tsukiyama-Kohara K, Kohara M, Matsumoto M, Seya T, Oshiumi H. Extracellular vesicles including exosomes regulate innate immune responses to hepatitis B virus infection. Frontiers in Immunology. 2016;**7**:335

[120] McLauchlan J, Addison C, Craigie MC, Rixon FJ. Noninfectious L-particles supply functions which can facilitate infection by HSV-1. Virology. 1992;**190**:682-688

[121] Rixon FJ, Addison C, McLauchlan J. Assembly of enveloped tegument structures (L particles) can occur independently of virion maturation in herpes simplex virus type 1-infected cells. Journal of General Virology. 1992;**73**:277-284

[122] Heilingloh CS, Kummer M, Mühl-Zürbes P, Drassner C, Daniel C, Klewer M, Steinkasserer A. L particles transmit viral proteins from herpes simplex virus 1-infected mature dendritic cells to uninfected bystander cells, inducing CD83 downmodulation. Journal of Virology. 2015;**89**:11046-11055

[123] Chen R, Zhao X, Wang Y, Xie Y, Liu J. Hepatitis B virus X protein is capable of down-regulating protein level of host antiviral protein APOBEC3G. Scientific Reports. 2017;**7**: 40783

[124] Bukong TN, Momen-Heravi F, Kodys K, Bala S, Szabo G. Exosomes from hepatitis C infected patients transmit HCV infection and contain replication competent viral RNA in complex with Ago2-miR122-HSP90. PLOS Pathogens. 2014;**10**:e1004424

[125] Sattentau Q. Avoiding the void: cell-to-cell spread of human viruses. Nature Reviews Microbiology. 2008;**6**:815-826

[126] Brimacombe CL, Grove J, Meredith LW, Hu K, Syder AJ, Flores MV, Timpe JM, Krieger SE, Baumert TF, Tellinghuisen TL, Wong-Staal F, Balfe P, McKeating JA. Neutralizing antibody-resistant hepatitis C virus cell-to-cell transmission. Journal of Virology. 2011;**85**:596-605

[127] Li J, Liu K, Liu Y, Xu Y, Zhang F, Yang H, Liu J, Pan T, Chen J, Wu M, Zhou X, Yuan Z. Exosomes mediate the cell-to-cell transmission of IFN-α-induced antiviral activity. Nature Immunology. 2013;**14**:793-803

[128] Temme S, Eis-Hübinger AM, McLellan AD, Koch N. The herpes simplex virus-1 encoded glycoprotein B diverts HLA-DR into the exosome pathway. Journal of Immunology. 2010;**184**:236-243

[129] Plazolles N, Humbert J-M, Vachot L, Verrier B, Hocke C, Halary F. Pivotal advance: The promotion of soluble DC-SIGN release by inflammatory signals and its enhancement of cytomegalovirus-mediated cis-infection of myeloid dendritic cells. Journal of Leukocyte Biology. 2011;**89**:329-342

[130] Arenaccio C, Anticoli S, Manfredi F, Chiozzini C, Olivetta E, Federico M. Latent HIV-1 is activated by exosomes from cells infected with either replication-competent or defective HIV-1. Retrovirology. 2015;**12**:87

[131] Sampey GC, Saifuddin M, Schwab A, Barclay R, Punya S, Chung M-C, Hakami RM, Zadeh MA, Lepene B, Klase ZA, El-Hage N, Young M, Iordanskiy S, Kashanchi F. Exosomes from HIV-1-infected cells stimulate production of Pro-inflammatory cytokines through Trans-activating response (TAR) RNA. Journal of Biological Chemistry. 2016;**291**:1251-1266

[132] Dhib-Jalbut S, Hoffman PM, Yamabe T, Sun D, Xia J, Eisenberg H, Bergey G, Ruscetti FW. Extracellular human T-cell lymphotropic virus type I Tax protein induces cytokine production in adult human microglial cells. Annals of Neurology. 1994;**36**:787-790

[133] Shembade N, Harhaj EW. Role of post-translational modifications of HTLV-1 Tax in NF-κB activation. World Journal of Biological Chemistry. 2010;**1**:13-20

[134] Honegger A, Schilling D, Bastian S, Sponagel J, Kuryshev V, Sültmann H, Scheffner M, Hoppe-Seyler K, Hoppe-Seyler F. Dependence of intracellular and exosomal microRNAs on viral E6/E7 oncogene expression in HPV-positive tumor cells. PLOS Pathogens. 2015;**11**:e1004712

[135] Feng Z, Hensley L, McKnight KL, Hu F, Madden V, Ping L, Jeong S-H, Walker C, Lanford RE, Lemon SM. A pathogenic picornavirus acquires an envelope by hijacking cellular membranes. Nature. 2013;**496**:367-371

[136] Yang Y, Han Q, Hou Z, Zhang C, Tian Z, Zhang J. Exosomes mediate hepatitis B virus (HBV) transmission and NK-cell dysfunction. Cellular & Molecular Immunology. 2017;**14**(5):465-475

[137] Dreux M, Garaigorta U, Boyd B, Décembre E, Chung J, Whitten-Bauer C, Wieland S, Chisari FV. Short-Range exosomal transfer of viral RNA from infected cells to plasmacytoid dendritic cells triggers innate immunity. Cell Host & Microbe. 2012;**12**:558-570

[138] Ahsan NA, Sampey GC, Lepene B, Akpamagbo Y, Barclay RA, Iordanskiy S, Hakami RM, Kashanchi F. Presence of viral RNA and proteins in exosomes from cellular clones resistant to rift valley fever virus infection. Frontiers in Microbiology. 2016;**7**:139

Chapter 5

Exosomes as the Promising Biomarker for Epstein-Barr Virus (EBV)-Associated Cancers

Sin-Yeang Teow and Suat-Cheng Peh

Additional information is available at the end of the chapter

http://dx.doi.org/10.5772/intechopen.69532

Abstract

Exosomes are microvesicles with sizes ranging from 50 to 150 nm. These small vesicles are known to morphologically and functionally resemble virus particles from human immunodeficiency virus type I (HIV-I) and human T-lymphotropic virus type I (HTLV-I). The function of exosomes is to mainly mediate cell-to-cell communication by exchanging various macromolecules including proteins, lipids and nucleic acids in diverse cellular processes. Due to its size and structural simplicity, the transfer of pathogenic or virulent cellular factors across the cells mediated by exosomes is more efficient, hence facilitating the dissemination of viral infections and cancer diseases. The pathogenic role of exosomes in various cancers such as lung and breast, and their potentials as biomarkers have been previously studied, yet limited information is known for Epstein-Barr virus (EBV)-associated cancers. In this chapter, we discuss current evidences that support the pathogenic roles of exosomes in EBV-related cancers and their potentials as biomarkers in cancer diagnostics and therapy response. Here, we also highlight the potential challenges in the development of exosome-based biomarkers for clinical application.

Keywords: EBV, exosomes, cancer, biomarker, nasopharyngeal carcinoma, diagnostics, therapy

1. Introduction

Exosomes are microvesicles that play major roles in cell-to-cell communication. These small vesicles have nano-scaled size, resembling the size of HIV-1 particles. Indeed, several reports have highlighted the similarity between exosomes and HIV-1 particles in terms of structure and functions [1, 2]. Biological roles of exosomes in HIV-1 pathogenesis have been extensively reviewed and the implication of the pathogenic exosomes depends highly on the contents that they carry [3, 4]. The functions of exosomes in other viral infections, such as hepatitis

C virus (HCV), herpes simplex virus (HSV) and so on, have also been demonstrated [5, 6]. In addition to viral diseases, exosomes have also been reported to play critical roles in cancer pathogenesis, including those in glioma, lymphoma, colorectal carcinoma, melanoma, ovarian and breast cancers [7, 8]. However, little is known for the function of exosomes derived from tumour viruses or oncoviruses such as HTLV-1, EBV and human papilloma viruses (HPV) in virus spreading as well as oncovirus-driven tumour development and dissemination. Among all, EBV is the most common infection and it infects more than 90% of human adult population globally [9]. Cumulative findings demonstrated that EBV infection is associated with various lymphoid and epithelial malignancies, including nasopharyngeal carcinoma (NPC), Burkitt's lymphoma (BL), gastric carcinoma (GC), Hodgkin's lymphoma (HL) and Non-Hodgkin's lymphoma [9, 10]. Similarly, EBV has also been reported to contribute to breast and cervical cancers [11, 12]. **Figure 1** summarizes the cancers that are associated with EBV infection, and percent association with EBV is depicted in a form of pyramid.

Exosomes are ubiquitously present in almost all biological fluids, including urine, plasma, saliva, ascites, breast milk, semen, bronchoalveolar lavage liquid, amniotic fluid and cerebrospinal fluid [4–7]. They are secreted from various cell types such as dendritic cells (DCs), macrophages, T cells, B cells and cancerous cells [4–7]. The omnipresence of exosomes makes them the ideal targets for cancer diagnostics and anti-cancer therapy. However, it remains to be seen whether exosomes from different sources present similar pathogenic profiles and can be interchangeably targeted for diagnostics and therapeutic purposes. Exosomes generally have a density of 1.13–1.21 g/mL [13]. They are surrounded by a lipid bilayer and they are enriched with macromolecules such as lipids (e.g. cholesterol and glycosphingolipids), carbohydrates (e.g. high mannose and complex N-linked glycans), proteins (e.g. tetraspanins CD9, CD63 and CD81, MHC molecules, Rabs, actin, alix, HSP70 and TSG101) and nucleic acids (e.g. DNAs, mRNAs and miRNAs) [14, 15]. While EBV infection is highly associated

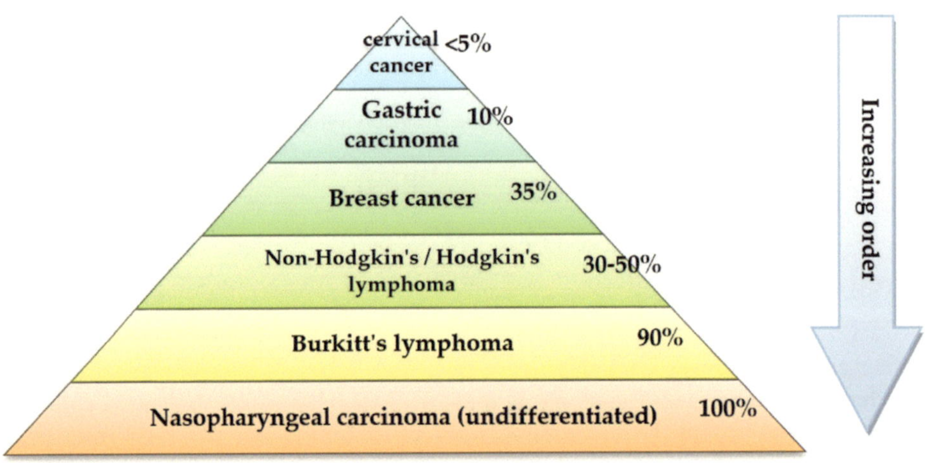

Figure 1. Association of EBV infection with virus-associated cancers. The association of EBV and cancers is represented by the above pyramid in a rising order from top to bottom. Almost 100% of undifferentiated NPC cases are associated with EBV infection while cervical cancer has been reported to be linked with EBV infection, but to the least extent with about less than 5% of total cases.

with a plethora of cancer diseases, it is strikingly surprising that only a few studies have been carried out to investigate the role of EBV-derived exosomes in cancer development and progression. This chapter aims to summarize current findings that demonstrate the biological functions of EBV-derived exosomes in the cancer pathogenesis. We also attempt to discuss the potentials of using EBV-derived exosomes as diagnostic biomarkers and to target these exosomes in anti-cancer therapy, while reviewing the challenges entailed in the above efforts.

2. Pathogenic roles of exosomes in EBV-associated cancers

Exosomes are originated from cellular endosomes, whereby the inward budding takes place on endosomal multivesicular bodies (MVBs) to form intraluminal vesicles (ILVs) [5, 6]. The subsequent molecular event then determines whether ILVs enter lysosomal degradation pathway or are being secreted out from the producer cells in the form of exosomes upon the fusion of MVB membrane with the plasma membrane [5, 6]. **Figure 2** illustrates these processes that involve the budding of endosomes, formation of EBV pathogenic factors-loaded exosomes and the delivery of the pathogenic exosomes to the target cells. The biogenesis of exosomes has been previously reviewed in great depth [14, 15], and these findings are important to enhance our understandings towards the function of exosomes in multiple cellular processes especially in cancer pathogenesis. The role of EBV-derived exosomes in EBV-associated cancers has been partly discussed in previous reviews [5, 8], but the proteins or genes involved and the underlying mechanisms have not been clearly illustrated. In this section, we will discuss the pathogenic roles of the contents in EBV-derived exosomes such as latent membrane proteins (LMPs), mRNAs and miRNAs in contributing to the EBV-associated cancers.

2.1. Exosomal latent membrane proteins (LMPs)

Latent membrane proteins (LMPs) are oncogenic proteins that are highly associated with cancer pathogenesis particularly in HL and NPC. There are two types of LMPs: LMP1, and LMP2 that consists of LMP2A and LMP2B. Each of these oncogenic proteins has distinct function in EBV-related human cancers [16, 17]. For instances, LMP1, which is a viral mimic of tumour necrosis factor receptor (TNFR) family member CD40, has been reported to activate a cascade of oncogenic signalling pathways such as nuclear factor kappa B (NF-κB), phosphatidylinositol-4,5-bisphosphate 3-kinase (PI3K) and c-Jun N-terminal kinases (JNKs) in EBV-associated cancers [10, 16, 17]. On the other hand, LMP2 plays central roles in maintaining viral latency in EBV-infected B cells as well as inducing transformation and migration of EBV-infected cells [10, 16, 17]. Whether or not the functions of cell-associated LMPs are fully retained in the exosomal LMPs, it remains to be proven. The development of the EBV-related cancers is associated with three EBV latency types based on the expression of EBV proteins (i.e. LMP1, LMP2 and Epstein-Barr virus nuclear antigen-1, EBNA1). Latency type I, which is usually observed in BL and GC, consistently displays strong expression of EBNA1 [17, 18]. Latency type II, on the other hand, results in the expression of LMP1, LMP2 and EBNA1 as seen in HL and NPC, whereas in latency type III, all latent proteins/antigens are expressed in the course of acquired immune deficiency syndrome (AIDS)-related lymphomas and lymphoblastoid

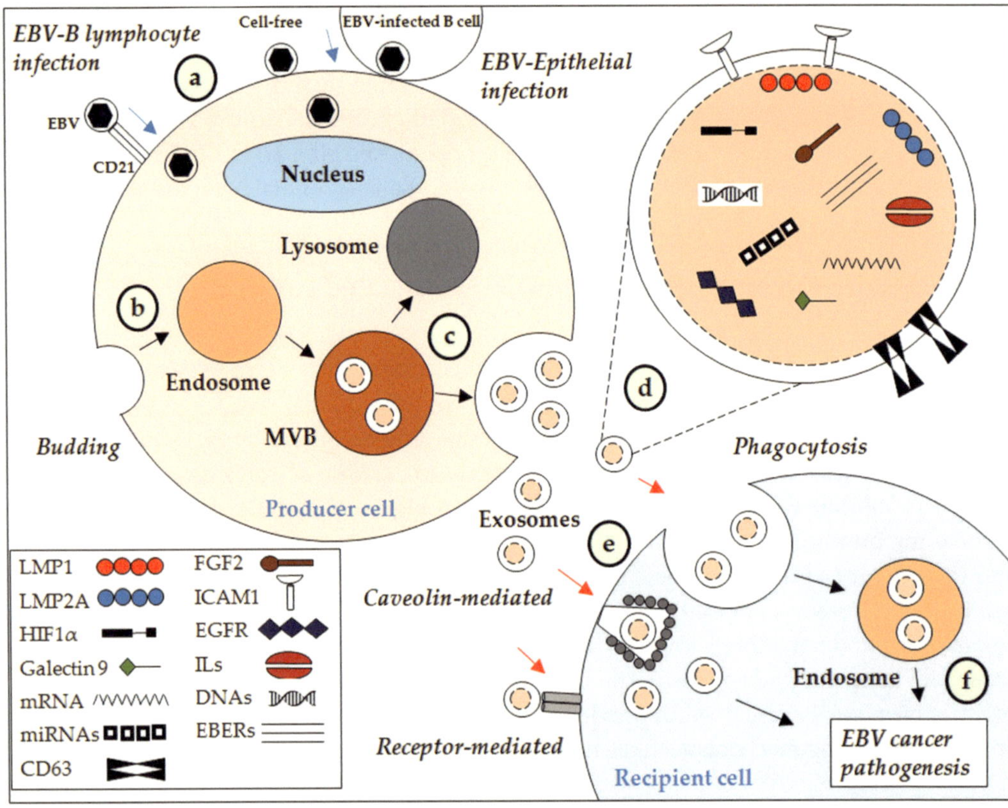

Figure 2. Generation of exosomes in EBV-infected cells and delivery of EBV pathogenic factors-enriched exosomes to recipient cells. (a) EBV infects B cells through viral glycoproteins/CD21 interaction, whereas EBV could infect epithelial cells either through cell-free manner or cell-to-cell contact mediated by infected B cells. (b) Exosomes are generated from the inward budding of endosomes, which then forms MVBs followed by ILVs. (c) ILVs are then either degraded by lysosomes or released from the producer cells extracellularly as exosomes. (d) Owing to the overexpression of EBV proteins/genes in the infected cell, exosomes are loaded with these pathogenic factors. (e) These exosomes are then delivered to the neighbouring cells via phagocytosis, receptor- or caveolin-mediated endocytosis. (f) The pathogenic factors are released from the EBV-derived exosomes, which then contribute to the cancer pathogenesis.

cell lines (LCLs) [17, 18]. Of note, the LMPs-carrying exosomes have been previously shown to be secreted by EBV-infected cells particularly the NPC cells [19–21].

So far, only a few studies have shown the involvement of exosomal LMP1 in activating various oncogenic pathways in EBV-associated cancers unlike those in the case of cell-derived LMP1 [16, 17]. Current findings suggest that exosome-derived LMP-1 plays central roles in attenuating the immune response in both EBV infection and the development and progression of EBV cancers [20, 22, 23]. For instances, the LMP1- and galectin 9-containing exosomes derived from EBV-infected LCLs and NPC cells have been found to inhibit infiltrating T-lymphocyte activation and proliferation through an action mediated by the conserved trans-membrane domain of LMP1 [20]. This consequently resulted in the immune escape of tumour cells, and hence promoting the cancer growth and progression [24]. Exosomes containing LMP1 and HIFα have also been demonstrated to induce tumour invasion in NPC [19]. Moreover, LMP1 was shown to promote the expression of fibroblasts growth factor 2 (FGF2) and along with the LMP1, FGF2 was excreted from the tumour cells via Na(+)/K(+)-ATPase-dependent exosomal pathway [25]. Notably, FGF2 is an important angiogenic factor in tumour invasion and it has been recently shown that FGF2 can be targeted by miR-16 to inhibit in cell proliferation and invasion in NPC [26]. However, whether or not the LMP1-induced exosome-derived FGF2 secretion is implicated in the EBV-associated cancers, particularly in the aspect of tumour metastasis warrants further investigations.

On top of the immunosuppressive and potentially invasive roles of exosomal LMP1, expression of intercellular adhesion molecule 1 (ICAM1) or CD54 was also up-regulated by exosomal LMP1 [21]. Notably, overexpression of ICAM1 is generally seen in various types of EBV-related cancers such as NPC, GC and NHL [27–29]. Similarly, exosomal LMP1 also induced epidermal growth factor receptor (EGFR) expression [30] which is another important receptor that modulates a cascade of oncogenic signalling pathways such as mitogen-activated protein kinase (MAPK), c-Jun N terminal kinase (JNK), phosphatidylinositol 3 kinase (PI3K) and nuclear factor kappa-beta (NF-κB) in EBV cancers [31, 32]. In line with of the role of exosomal LMP1 in EGFR-related pathways, Meckes and co-workers also demonstrated that exosomal LMP1 activated Extracellular signal-regulated kinase (ERK) and v-Akt murine thymoma viral oncogene homolog (AKT) signalling pathways in the target cells [30]. This finding suggests that the transfer of oncogenic LMP1 via exosomal pathway may modulate the growth of neighbouring cells, hence contributing to the cellular transformation of cancer cells.

Interestingly, exosomal LMP1 is also found to interact with tetraspanin CD63, a common marker of exosomes. This interaction facilitates the former to escape lysosomal degradation [33] which may result in enhanced oncogenicity of exosomal LMP1. In addition, the level of LMP1 is highly correlated with CD63 expression [19]. This suggests that LMP1 may upregulate the exosomal secretion, hence promoting the EBV-associated cancers [19]. As summarized in **Table 1**, cumulative findings suggest that exosomal LMP1 promotes the growth and progression of EBV-associated cancers. While the cell-associated or intracellular LMP1 plays multiple roles in EBV latent infection and cancer pathogenesis particularly by modulating NF-κB, PI3K/AKT, MAPK and JAK/STAT pathways [31, 32], future investigations are warranted to demonstrate whether the exosomal LMP1 similarly carries these tumorigenic functions and pathogenic effects in EBV-associated cancers.

As compared with LMP1, the role and function of exosomal LMP2A/2B in EBV-associated cancers are less understood. Incorporation of LMP2 into exosomes has been previously observed and these exosomes were released and taken by recipient cells [34, 35–37]. Several studies have provided insights on the mechanism of exosomal LMP2 secretion. Ikeda and Longnecker demonstrated that cholesterol depletion via methyl-beta-cyclodextrin (MCD) depletion can increase exosomal secretion of LMP2A, indicating the inverse dependency between the release of LMP2A-carrying exosomes and cholesterol level [35]. In another study, the interaction between LMP2A and endocytic adapter proteins, Amphiphysin 1 and 2 was found to be essential in order for LMP2A to accumulate into exosomes [38]. However, no further study has been done to investigate the pathogenic role of Amphiphysin proteins on EBV-associated cancers. Future investigations are required to uncover the pathogenic role of exosomal LMP2 in these cancers.

Exosomal content	Pathogenic effect	Reference
LMP1 & HIF1α	Promotion of tumour invasion	[19]
LMP1 & Galectin 9	Immunosuppression of T lymphocytes	[20]
LMP1 & ICAM1	Induction of ICAM1 expression by LMP1 Modulation of multiple oncogenic pathways	[21]
LMP1 & FGF2	Induction of FGF2 expression by LMP1 Potential driver of tumour invasion	[25]
LMP1 & EGFR	Induction of EGFR expression by LMP1 Modulation of multiple oncogenic pathways	[30]
LMP1 & CD63	Increased secretion of exosomal LMP1	[33]
LMP2A & Amphiphysin	Increased secretion of exosomal LMP2A	[38]
BHRF1-3 miRNA	Detected in the EBV-infected cells and transferable via exosomes	[43]
miR-BART15-3p	Detected in EBV-infected cells and transferable via exosomes to corresponding cells	[44]
hsa-miR-24-3p hsa-miR-891p hsa-miR-106a-5p hsa-miR-20a-5p hsa-miR-1908	Inhibition of T-cell proliferation and differentiation Induction of Treg cells Increased pro-inflammatory cytokine expression Regulation of MARK1 signaling pathway	[45]
EBV latent phase mRNAs	Potential expression of LMP1, LMP2, EBNA1, and EBNA2 in recipient cells upon taking up these exosomes	[46]
EBER1 and EBER2	Detected in the EBV-infected cells and transferable via exosomes	[47]
CCL20	Enhanced Treg recruitment and expansion	[22]
dUTPase	Induction of NK-κB activation and pro-inflammatory cytokine secretion	[48]
IFI16, caspase-1, IL-1β, IL-18, IL-33	Enrichment of caspase-1 resulted in the secretion of active immune-modulatory cytokines	[49]

Table 1. Potential pathogenic roles of exosomes in EBV-associated cancers.

2.2. Exosomal RNAs

Cancer-derived exosomes carry RNAs particularly miRNAs that are implicated in cancer pathogenesis such as in breast and colorectal cancers [39, 40]. In EBV-related cancers, the pathogenic role of RNAs such as miRNAs, mRNAs and Epstein-Barr virus-encoded small RNAs (EBERs) has drawn considerable attention in the past few years [17, 41]. miRNAs are non-coding RNAs that modulate multiple cellular processes, including the promotion of tumourigenesis via a cascade of signalling pathways [41]. They are small molecules with an approximate size of 22 nucleotides [41]. The mature miRNA functions by interacting with the target mRNA and block their activities by repressing the translation. The effects of miRNAs have been implicated in various EBV-associated cancers such as NPC, GC and BL [17, 41, 42]. However, the tumorigenic role of exosomal miRNAs is underexplored in EBV-related cancers as opposed to the cellular miRNAs.

There are substantial findings supporting the notion that oncogenic miRNA-carrying exosomes may play pathogenic roles in EBV-associated cancers [21, 30, 43]. For instances, BHRF1-3 miRNA has been shown to be secreted from the EBV-infected cells and they retained their cellular function upon delivery to the recipient cells [43]. Choi and colleagues demonstrated that the miR-BART15-3p could be detected in EBV-associated exosomes and its expression level was 2 to 16-fold higher in the exosomes compared with the cellular level in GC cells [44], hence suggesting its potential tumorigenic role. On the other hand, Ye and group showed that the exosomal miRNAs promoted the tumour progression by modulating multiple cellular processes in NPC [45] (**Table 1**). Further studies are required to investigate and validate their roles in promoting EBV-derived cancers. The occurrence of exosomes carrying mRNAs encoding for oncogenic EBV proteins such as LMP1, LMP2, EBNA1 and EBNA2 [46, 47] as well as EBERs has also been documented (**Figure 1**). While the functions of these RNAs in the EBV-infected cancer cells are well-described, whether or not the exosomal RNAs are transferable to the recipient cells and exert their tumorigenic effects remains a question.

2.3. Other exosomal pathogenic factors

In addition to EBV-associated proteins/genes such as LMPs, EBERs, EBV-related miRNAs and mRNAs, exosomes related to EBV-associated cancers may also contain other endogenous proteins that potentially promote cancer progression such as transcription factor Galectin-9 [20], EGFR [30], HIF1α [19], ICAM1 [21], FGF2 [25], chemokine (C-C motif) ligand 20 (CCL20) [22], dUTPase [48] and interleukins (ILs)/caspase 1/interferon-inducible protein 16 (IFI16) [49] (**Table 1**).

Mrizak and co-workers demonstrated that CCL20-containing exosomes recruited the CD25+FOXP3+ Treg cells and enhanced their expansion in NPC [22]. The involvement of these exosomes in the Treg interaction may therefore support immune evasion in NPC. In the case of dUTPase enzyme, up-regulated expression of this enzyme has been observed in the exosomes derived from the EBV-positive Burkitt's lymphoma cell line, Raji. These enzymes are found to induce the cytokine release from DCs and PBMCs, which may activate the NF-κB pathway [48].

Interestingly, exosomes derived from the Raji cells and other EBV-infected cell lines are also enriched with various immune modulators such as IFI16, cleaved caspase-1, IL-1β, IL-18 and IL-33 [49]. The presence of these proteins in these exosomes may suggest that EBV utilizes the host exosome pathway in immune escape of tumour hence contributing to the EBV-associated cancer progression.

3. Exosomes as biomarkers

We have discussed the tumorigenic role of exosomes in EBV-associated cancers in previous section. Since these exosomes carry a great variety of pathogenic molecules (**Figure 2**), they can be potentially used for diagnostic and/or prognostic markers in the EBV-related cancers. Indeed, several reports have highlighted the potentials of employing exosomes as the biomarkers in various cancers [50, 51], and the exosome-containing miRNAs are the most popular cancer diagnostic markers out of all [52, 53]. There have been several lines of evidences suggesting that EBV oncoproteins can be targeted for cancer diagnostics. For instances, Houali and colleagues showed that both EBV oncoproteins, LMP1 and BARF1, could be detected in serum and saliva of NPC patients, and the secreted LMP1 was highly associated with exosome-like vesicles [54]. Both EBV oncoproteins were presented with high mitogenic activity that supported their implication in oncogenic development of NPC. The fact that exosomes are abundantly expressed in patient serum and saliva further support the potential of using the oncoprotein-enriched exosomes for cancer diagnostics [3–5]. Similarly, Mao and co-workers also highlighted the potential of LMP1 and LMP2A as the prognostic markers for extranodal NK/T-cell lymphoma (ENKTL) patients [55]. LMP1 and LMP2A were overexpressed in ENKTL tumours and they significantly correlated with the patients' overall survival. However, whether or not the exosomal LMP1 and LMP2A have the similar values for prognosis remain to be seen.

In addition, other pathogenic factors that are enriched in EBV exosomes such as EBV DNAs, EBV mRNAs and EBV miRNAs have also been shown to be potential biomarkers for EBV cancer diagnosis [56–59] (**Table 2**). Using quantitative PCR (qPCR), Yip and colleagues showed that high-EBV DNAs could be detected in plasma/serum of NPC patients at late stages of disease and the viral loads were associated with poor survival or frequent relapse in NPC patients [56, 59]. On the other hand, Stevens and colleagues demonstrated that the EBV DNA load measurement might have limited value as the diagnostic marker for NPC as the viral load did not reflect the intact tumour cells [56, 59]. Hence, they recommended to combine circulating EBV DNA measurement and EBV serology to increase the diagnostic sensitivity. The same group also showed that the combination of EBV DNA and BARF1 mRNAs detection from patients' nasopharyngeal brushings could be a good non-invasive method for

Exosomal target	Source/sample	Cancer type	Reference
LMP1	Serum, saliva, tumour	Lymphoma, NPC	[54, 55]
LMP2A	Tumour	Lymphoma	[55]
BARF1	Serum, saliva	NPC	[54]
EBV DNAs	Cell lines, tumour, NP brushing, serum/plasma	NPC	[56, 57, 59]
EBV mRNAs	Cell lines, tumour, NP brushing, serum	NPC	[57, 59]
EBV miRNAs	Cell lines, plasma	NPC	[58]
Galectin	Tumour	NPC	[65]
EGFR	Tumour	Prostate cancer*	[61]
HIF1α	Tumour	Breast cancer	[60]

*Not EBV-associated cancer.

Table 2. Potential exosomal target for prognostic/diagnostic biomarker development in EBV cancers.

http://dx.doi.org/10.5772/intechopen.69532

NPC diagnosis [57]. On the other hand, Zhang and co-workers showed that EBV miRNAs (miR-BART7 and miR-BART13) can serve as important biomarkers for NPC diagnosis and prediction of treatment efficacy [58]. The potential prognostic value of EGFR and HIF1α has been previously demonstrated in breast and prostate cancers [60, 61]. It would be interesting if these proteins can also be used as prognostic markers for EBV-related cancers. However, this requires further investigations. While circulating EBV DNAs, mRNAs, miRNAs and other components in serum/plasma is useful for EBV-related cancer diagnostics, more efforts should be focused in discriminating the diagnostics values of cell- and exosome-derived nucleic acids.

More interestingly, exosomes have shown to protect their cargoes from degradation. For instance, it has been shown that the mRNAs and miRNAs encapsulated in exosomes are protected from RNAses [62]. They are more stable and can be stably employed as diagnostic biomarkers. Recent advances in methods have also made the exosome isolation from various biofluids simpler, more straightforward, and with better quality and yield [63, 64]. The EBV proteins/genes that can potentially be developed into diagnostic markers are summarized in **Table 2**.

4. Exosomes as predictive markers for therapy response

Pathogenic exosomes have been previously linked to the treatment failure of cancers [65, 66]. As exosomes exhibit pathogenic effects on tumour formation and progression, the oncogenic activity of exosomes can be intervened by blocking the production/release of the exosomes or the specific exosomal proteins/genes. **Figure 2** summarizes the pathogenic and tumorigenic factors derived from the EBV exosomes and the potential targets for anti-cancer therapy development. In fact, there have been studies showing that EBV-associated proteins and nucleic acids (e.g. DNA, mRNA and miRNA) can be targeted for anti cancer therapy development particularly in NPC [67–70]. For instance, various strategies, such as cell-based immunotherapy, antibody-based and drug-based therapies, have been developed against EBV LMPs in NPC [68]. Similarly, Cao and colleagues also showed that DNAzyme resulted in significant tumour regression by targeting and cleaving off the LMP1 mRNA from NPC patients [67]. Other non-EBV tumour-promoting but LMP-associated proteins that could be targeted in NPC are EGFR [71, 72] and vascular endothelial growth factor (VEGF) [73, 74]. In addition, targeting the whole exosome has also been shown to be a potent therapeutic strategy for cancer therapy [66, 75]. However, the potential of developing these pathogenic proteins derived from tumour-associated exosomes into the therapy is unclear and further investigations are required.

As abovementioned, exosomes also contribute to the immune evasion of cancer cells [20, 22, 23]. For example, the galectin-9-containing exosomes have been shown to inhibit the proliferation and induce apoptosis of EBV-specific T cell, hence preventing the T cell-mediated recognition and killing of these cancer cells [20, 23]. Therefore, blocking these exosomes may restore the functions of immune cells to act and kill the cancer cells together with a plethora of other active tumour-killing activities. It can be envisioned that the development of a therapeutic strategy blocking the galectin-9 or other proteins from oncogenic exosomes may restore the immune surveillance. Over the past few years, considerable work has also been done on targeting the whole exosomes rather than targeting the specific proteins [76, 77]. The exosomal removal using a modified kidney dialysis system has also been proposed to bring this therapeutic approach to the clinics [76]. These findings suggest that diminishing or eliminating the tumorigenic exosomes may be a good therapeutic approach to reverse the exosome-mediated cancer progression, particularly in the aspect of immune dysregulation.

5. Challenges and limitations

The facts that exosomes are ubiquitous and can be detected in most of the biofluids give advantages to the development of diagnostics biomarkers. Several studies have also demonstrated that biologically functional and intact exosomes could be isolated from human plasma/serum [63, 64]. Moreover, the isolation/purification method of high-quality and quantity exosomes from body fluids has greatly improved in the past few years [63, 64]. Hence, the development of exosome-targeting diagnostic biomarker has high potential and can be developed into an important liquid biopsy-based diagnostic test for cancers in future. However, several considerations need to be taken into account to ensure the success of biomarker and therapy development.

Sensitivity and specificity are important criteria for cancer biomarker development. While exosomes containing EBV-associated contents (e.g. mRNAs, miRNAs, LMPs, galectin 9 etc.) have tumour-promoting and pathogenic properties and are expressed during the disease development (**Table 1**), they are not specific to particular type of cancer of which they could contribute to such as NPC, GC, BL and so on (**Figure 1**). Before a specific exosomal target is discovered for each EBV-related cancer, other non-invasive tests such as cancer antigen screening and magnetic resonance imaging (MRI) can be carried out simultaneously to enhance the diagnostic outcome in terms of cancer specificity. Furthermore, the expression of some target protein/gene in the patients may highly depend on the disease state. The expression may be too low to be detected or undetected at all during the early stage of cancer, hence the sensitivity may be the issue. On top of that, the quality and quantity of the pathogenic exosomes can be a challenge for diagnostic biomarker development even though it has been shown that high quality of exosomes could be detected from cancer patients [63, 64]. This will highly rely on the method used for the exosome isolation/purification for the diagnostic purpose, and it is extremely important to ensure the high consistency and reproducibility of the test.

As an important therapeutic target, EBV proteins/nucleic acids can be targeted for tumour regression as described in the previous section. Exosomes play important roles in cell-cell communication mainly by regulating cellular processes, hence complete removal of exosomes is not a feasible therapeutic strategy as it will affect the well-being of other normal cells or cellular processes under a normal condition [7, 14]. Hence, it is important to specifically target only the exosomes enriched with the pathogenic factors without affecting the biological activities of existing exosomes. In addition, the exosomal contents may largely vary and are heterogeneous depending on the sources or origins [7, 14]. This may be another challenge especially the targeted exosomes are from the patient's body fluids that may be derived from a diverse range of cells. Furthermore,

Purpose	Potential issue	Note
Diagnostic biomarker development	Specificity	Not specific to particular cancer type
	Sensitivity	No/low expression in early-stage cancer
	Quality	Inactive and not functional exosomal content
	Quantity	Low yield of the pathogenic exosome or protein/gene
Anti-cancer therapy development	Toxicity	Off-target effect against all functional exosomes
	Heterogeneity	Contain multiple types of functional protein/gene
	Dose and course	Wide in range due to the personalized differences
	Delivery	Therapeutics may not reach the ubiquitous exosomes
	Bioavailability	Therapeutics may be degraded before reaching to the targets

Table 3. Potential challenges for the development of exosome-targeted cancer diagnostics and anti-cancer therapy.

some potential targets may be scarcely expressed or not at all in the targeted exosomes which will hinder the efficiency to target exosomes for any anti-cancer therapy. Other considerations include the dosage of exosome-targeting drugs that may vary from one to another, the delivery system for targeting exosomes, the bioavailability/stability of the delivered therapeutic molecules and the treatment course. Further works are required to evaluate the clinical safety of exosome-targeting treatment strategy. **Table 3** summarizes the potential challenges during the development of diagnostic marker and therapy by targeting the exosomes in EBV cancers.

6. Conclusion

EBV-derived exosomes play seminal roles in the pathogenesis of EBV-associated cancers especially in NPC. Cumulative findings suggest that EBV-exosomes may be ideal targets for the development of diagnostic/prognostic markers and anti-cancer therapy. However, several issues need to be taken into account during the development as abovementioned. As limited studies have been carried out, more investigations are required to further validate the feasibility of targeting the pathogenic EBV exosomes for clinical diagnosis of EBV cancers. Current findings also suggest that the targeted exosomes could be developed into vaccines for EBV infections to reduce the EBV-induced cancers.

Acknowledgements

We like to thank Sunway Internal Research Grant (INTM-2017-SIDS-SIHD-01) and Rewarding Research Output (RRO) (INT-RRO-2017-095) from Sunway University and National Cancer Council Malaysia (MAKNA) Cancer Research Award (CRA) 2016 (EXT-SIDS-SIHD-MAKNA-2017-01) for partly supporting this work.

Author details

Sin-Yeang Teow[1]* and Suat-Cheng Peh[1,2]

*Address all correspondence to: ronaldt@sunway.edu.my

1 Sunway Institute for Healthcare Development (SIHD), Sunway University, Selangor, Malaysia

2 Anatomical Pathology Department, Sunway Medical Centre, Selangor, Malaysia

References

[1] Izquierdo-Useros N, Puertas M, Borràs F, Blanco J, Martinez-Picado J. Exosomes and retroviruses: The chicken or the egg?. Cellular Microbiology. 2010;**13**(1):10-17. DOI: 10.1111/j.1462-5822.2010.01542.x

[2] Booth A, Fang Y, Fallon J, Yang J, Hildreth J, Gould S. Exosomes and HIV Gag bud from endosome-like domains of the T cell plasma membrane. The Journal of Cell Biology. 2006;**172**(6):923-935. DOI: 10.1083/jcb.200508014

[3] Madison M, Okeoma C. Exosomes: Implications in HIV-1 pathogenesis. Viruses. 2015;**7**(7): 4093-4118. DOI: 10.3390/v7072810

[4] Teow S, Nordin A, Ali S, Khoo A. Exosomes in human immunodeficiency virus type I pathogenesis: Threat or opportunity?. Advances in Virology. 2016;**2016**:1-8. DOI: 10.1155/2016/9852494

[5] Meckes D, Raab-Traub N. Microvesicles and viral infection. Journal of Virology. 2011;**85**(24):12844-12854. DOI: 10.1128/JVI.05853-11

[6] Schwab A, Meyering S, Lepene B, Iordanskiy S, van Hoek M, Hakami R, et al. Extracellular vesicles from infected cells: Potential for direct pathogenesis. Frontiers in Microbiology. 2015;**6**:1132. DOI: 10.3389/fmicb.2015.01132

[7] Zhang X, Yuan X, Shi H, Wu L, Qian H, Xu W. Exosomes in cancer: Small particle, big player. Journal of Hematology & Oncology. 2015;**8**:83. DOI: 10.1186/s13045-015-0181-x

[8] Yang C, Robbins P. The roles of tumor-derived exosomes in cancer pathogenesis. Clinical and Developmental Immunology. 2011;**2011**:1-11. DOI: 10.1155/2011/842849

[9] Niedobitek G, Meru N, Delecluse H. Epstein-Barr virus infection and human malignancies. International Journal of Experimental Pathology. 2008;**82**(3):149-170. DOI: 10.1111/j.1365-2613.2001.iep190.x

[10] Young L, Yap L, Murray P. Epstein–Barr virus: More than 50 years old and still providing surprises. Nature Reviews Cancer. 2016;**16**(12):789-802. DOI: 10.1038/nrc.2016.92

[11] Richardson A, Currie M, Robinson B, Morrin H, Phung Y, Pearson J, et al. Cytomegalovirus and Epstein-Barr virus in breast cancer. PLoS ONE. 2015;**10**(2):e0118989. DOI: 10.1371/journal.pone.0118989

[12] Shi Y, Peng S, Yang L, Chen X, Tao Y, Cao Y. Co-infection of Epstein-Barr virus and human papillomavirus in human tumorigenesis. Chinese Journal of Cancer. 2016;**35**:16. DOI: 10.1186/s40880-016-0079-1

[13] Thery C, Boussac M, Veron P, Ricciardi-Castagnoli P, Raposo G, Garin J, et al. Proteomic analysis of dendritic Cell-Derived exosomes: A secreted subcellular compartment distinct from apoptotic vesicles. The Journal of Immunology. 2001;**166**(12):7309-7318. DOI: 10.4049/jimmunol.166.12.7309

[14] Thery C, Zityogel L, Amigorena S. Exosomes: Composition, biogenesis and function. Nature Reviews Immunology. 2002;**2**(8):569-579. DOI: 10.1038/nri855

[15] Raposo G, Stoorvogel W. Extracellular vesicles: Exosomes, microvesicles, and friends. The Journal of Cell Biology. 2013;**200**(4):373-383. DOI: 10.1083/jcb.201211138

[16] Dawson C, Port R, Young L. The role of the EBV-encoded latent membrane proteins LMP1 and LMP2 in the pathogenesis of nasopharyngeal carcinoma (NPC). Seminars in Cancer Biology. 2012;**22**(2):144-153. DOI: 10.1016/j.semcancer

[17] Tsao S, Tsang C, To K, Lo K. The role of Epstein-Barr virus in epithelial malignancies. The Journal of Pathology. 2014;**235**(2):323-333. DOI: 10.1002/path.4448

[18] Ko Y. EBV and human cancer. Experimental & Molecular Medicine. 2015;**47**(1):e130. DOI: 10.1038/emm.2014.109

[19] Aga M, Bentz G, Raffa S, Torrisi M, Kondo S, Wakisaka N, et al. Exosomal HIF1α supports invasive potential of nasopharyngeal carcinoma-associated LMP1-positive exosomes. Oncogene. 2014;**33**(37):4613-4622. DOI: 10.1038/onc.2014.66

[20] Keryer-Bibens C, Pioche-Duricu C, Villemant C, Souquère S, Nishi N, Hirashima M, et al. Exosomes released by EBV-infected nasopharyngeal carcinoma cells convey the viral Latent Membrane Protein 1 and the immunomodulatory protein galectin 9. BMC Cancer. 2006;**6**:283. DOI: 10.1186/1471-2407-6-283

[21] Nanbo A, Kawanishi E, Yoshida R, Yoshiyama H. Exosomes derived from Epstein-Barr Virus-Infected cells are internalized via Caveola-Dependent endocytosis and promote phenotypic modulation in target cells. Journal of Virology. 2013;**87**(18):10334-10347. DOI: 10.1128/JVI.01310-13

[22] Mrizak D, Martin N, Barjon C, Jimenez-Pailhes A, Mustapha R, Niki T, et al. Effect of nasopharyngeal Carcinoma-Derived exosomes on human regulatory T cells. Journal of the National Cancer Institute. 2014;**107**(1):dju363. DOI: 10.1093/jnci/dju363

[23] Klibi J, Niki T, Riedel A, Pioche-Durieu C, Souquere S, Rubinstein E, et al. Blood diffusion and Th1-suppressive effects of galectin-9-containing exosomes released by Epstein-Barr virus-infected nasopharyngeal carcinoma cells. Blood. 2008;**113**(9):1957-1966. DOI: 10.1182/blood-2008-02-142596

[24] Dukers D, Meij P, Vervoort M, Vos W, Scheper R, Meijer C, et al. Direct immunosuppressive effects of EBV-Encoded latent membrane protein 1. The Journal of Immunology. 2000;**165**(2):663-670. DOI: 10.4049/jimmunol.165.2.663

[25] Ceccarelli S, Visco V, Raffa S, Wakisaka N, Pagano J, Torrisi M. Epstein-Barr virus latent membrane protein 1 promotes concentration in multivesicular bodies of fibroblast growth factor 2 and its release through exosomes. International Journal of Cancer. 2007;**121**(7):1494-1506. DOI: 10.1002/ijc.22844

[26] He Q, Rem X, Chen J, Li Y, Tang X, Wen X, et al. miR-16 targets fibroblast growth factor 2 to inhibit NPC cell proliferation and invasion via PI3K/AKT and MAPK signaling pathways. Oncotarget. 2016;**7**(3):3047-3058. DOI: 10.18632/oncotarget.6504

[27] Busson P, Zhang Q, Guillon J, Gregory C, Young L, Clausse B, et al. Elevated expression of ICAM1 (CD54) and minimal expression of LFA3 (CD58) in Epstein-Barr-virus-positive nasopharyngeal carcinoma cells. International Journal of Cancer. 1992;**50**(6):863-867. DOI: 10.1002/ijc.2910500605

[28] Jung W, Jang Y, Kim J, Park S, Park S, Kim S, et al. Expression of intercellular adhesion Molecule-1 and E-Selectin in gastric cancer and their clinical significance. Journal of Gastric Cancer. 2012;**12**(3):140. DOI: 10.5230/jgc.2012.12.3.140

[29] Terol M, Lopez-Guillermo A, Bosch F, Villamor N, Cid M, Rozman C, et al. Expression of the adhesion molecule ICAM-1 in non-Hodgkin's lymphoma: Relationship with tumor dissemination and prognostic importance. Journal of Clinical Oncology. 1998;**16**(1):35-40. DOI: 10.1016/0270-9139(95)90195-7

[30] Meckes D, Shair K, Marquitz A, Kung C, Edwards R, Raab-Traub N. Human tumor virus utilizes exosomes for intercellular communication. Proceedings of the National Academy of Sciences. 2010;**107**(47):20370-20375. DOI: 10.1073/pnas.1014194107

[31] Kung C, Meckes D, Raab-Traub N. Epstein-Barr virus LMP1 activates EGFR, STAT3, and ERK through effects on PKC. Journal of Virology. 2011;**85**(9):4399-4408. DOI: 10.1128/JVI.01703-10

[32] Tulalamba W, Janvilisri T. Nasopharyngeal carcinoma signaling pathway: An update on molecular biomarkers. International Journal of Cell Biology. 2012;**2012**:1-10. DOI: 10.1155/2012/594681

[33] Verweij F, van Eijndhoven M, Hopmans E, Vendrig T, Wurdinger T, Cahir-McFarland E, et al. LMP1 association with CD63 in endosomes and secretion via exosomes limits constitutive NF-κB activation. The EMBO Journal. 2011;**30**(11):2115-2129. DOI: 10.1038/emboj.2011.123

[34] Young L, Murray P. Epstein–Barr virus and oncogenesis: From latent genes to tumours. Oncogene. 2003;**22**(33):5108-5121. DOI: 10.1038/sj.onc.1206556

[35] Ikeda M, Longnecker R. Cholesterol is critical for Epstein-Barr virus latent membrane protein 2A trafficking and protein stability. Virology. 2007;**360**(2):461-468. DOI: 10.1016/j.virol.2006.10.046

[36] Schorey J, Cheng Y, Singh P, Smith V. Exosomes and other extracellular vesicles in host-pathogen interactions. EMBO Reports. 2014;**16**(1):24-43. DOI: 10.15252/embr.201439363

[37] Meckes D, Gunawardena H, Dekroon R, Heaton P, Edwards R, Ozgur S, et al. Modulation of B-cell exosome proteins by gamma herpesvirus infection. Proceedings of the National Academy of Sciences. 2013;**110**(31):E2925-E2933. DOI: 10.1073/pnas.1303906110

[38] Dergai O, Dergai M, Skrypkina I, Tsyba L, Yaruchik A, Rynditch A. Amphiphysin 1 and 2 interact with latent membrane protein 2A of Epstein-Barr virus and regulate its exosomal secretion. Biopolymers and Cell. 2012;**28**(3):234-238. DOI: 10.7124/bc.000054

[39] Zadran S, Remacle F, Levine R. miRNA and mRNA cancer signatures determined by analysis of expression levels in large cohorts of patients. Proceedings of the National Academy of Sciences. 2013;**110**(47):19160-19165. DOI: 10.1073/pnas.1316991110

[40] Cantini L, Isella C, Petti C, Picco G, Chiola S, Ficarra E, et al. MicroRNA–mRNA interactions underlying colorectal cancer molecular subtypes. Nature Communications. 2015;**6**:8878. DOI: 10.1038/ncomms9878

[41] Giudice A, D'Arena G, Crispo A, Tecce M, Nocerino F, Grimaldi M, et al. Role of viral miRNAs and epigenetic modifications in Epstein-Barr Virus-Associated gastric carcinogenesis. Oxidative Medicine and Cellular Longevity. 2016;**2016**:1-11. DOI: 10.1155/2016/6021934

[42] Spence T, Bruce J, Yip K, Liu F. MicroRNAs in nasopharyngeal carcinoma. Chinese Clinical Oncology. 2016;**5**(2):17. DOI: 10.21037/cco.2016.03.09

[43] Pegtel D, Cosmopoulos K, Thorley-Lawson D, van Eijndhoven M, Hopmans E, Lindenberg J, et al. Functional delivery of viral miRNAs via exosomes. Proceedings of the National Academy of Sciences. 2010;**107**(14):6328-6333. DOI: 10.1073/pnas.0914843107

[44] Choi H, Lee H, Kim S, Gho Y, Lee S. Epstein-Barr Virus-Encoded MicroRNA BART15-3p promotes cell apoptosis partially by targeting BRUCE. Journal of Virology. 2013;**87**(14):8135-8144. DOI: 10.1128/JVI.03159-12

[45] Ye S, Li Z, Luo D, Huang B, Chen Y, Zhang X, et al. Tumor-derived exosomes promote tumor progression and T-cell dysfunction through the regulation of enriched exosomal microRNAs in human nasopharyngeal carcinoma. Oncotarget. 2014;**5**(14):5439-5452. DOI: 10.18632/oncotarget.2118

[46] Canitano A, Venturi G, Borghi M, Ammendolia M, Fais S. Exosomes released in vitro from Epstein–Barr virus (EBV)-infected cells contain EBV-encoded latent phase mRNAs. Cancer Letters. 2013;**337**(2):193-199. DOI: 10.1016/j.canlet.2013.05.012

[47] Ahmed W, Philip P, Tariq S, Khan G. Epstein-Barr Virus-Encoded small RNAs (EBERs) are present in fractions related to exosomes released by EBV-Transformed cells. PLoS ONE. 2014;**9**(6):e99163. DOI: 10.1371/journal.pone.0099163

[48] Ariza M, Rivailler P, Glaser R, Chen M, Williams M. Epstein-Barr virus encoded dUTPase containing exosomes modulate innate and adaptive immune responses in human dendritic cells and peripheral blood mononuclear cells. PLoS ONE. 2013;**8**(7):e69827. DOI: 10.1371/journal.pone.0069827

[49] Ansari M, Singh V, Dutta S, Veettil M, Dutta D, Chikoti L, et al. Constitutive interferon-inducible protein 16-inflammasome activation during Epstein-Barr virus latency I, II, and III in B and epithelial cells. Journal of Virology. 2013;**87**(15):8606-8623. DOI: 10.1128/JVI.00805-13

[50] Lin J, Li J, Huang B, Liu J, Chen X, Chen X, et al. Exosomes: Novel biomarkers for clinical diagnosis. The Scientific World Journal. 2015;**2015**:1-8. DOI: 10.1155/2015/657086

[51] Munson P, Shukla A. Exosomes: Potential in cancer diagnosis and therapy. Medicines. 2015;**2**(4):310-327. DOI: 10.3390/medicines2040310

[52] Thind A, Wilson C. Exosomal miRNAs as cancer biomarkers and therapeutic targets. Journal of Extracellular Vesicles. 2016;**5**:31292. DOI: 10.3402/jev.v5.31292

[53] Nedaeinia R, Manian M, Jazayeri M, Ranjbar M, Salehi R, Sharifi M, et al. Circulating exosomes and exosomal microRNAs as biomarkers in gastrointestinal cancer. Cancer Gene Therapy. 2016. DOI: 10.1038/cgt.2016.77

[54] Houali K, Wang X, Shimizu Y, Djennaoui D, Nicholls J, Fiorini S, et al. A New Diagnostic marker for secreted Epstein-Barr virus encoded LMP1 and BARF1 oncoproteins in the serum and saliva of patients with nasopharyngeal carcinoma. Clinical Cancer Research. 2007;**13**(17):4993-5000. DOI: 10.1158/1078-0432.CCR-06-2945

[55] Mao Y, Zhang D, Zhu H, Lin H, Xiong L, Cao Q, et al. LMP1 and LMP2A are potential prognostic markers of extranodal NK/T-cell lymphoma, nasal type (ENKTL). Diagnostic Pathology. 2012;**7**(1):178. DOI: 10.1186/1746-1596-7-178

[56] Yip T, Ngan R, Fong A, Law S. Application of circulating plasma/serum EBV DNA in the clinical management of nasopharyngeal carcinoma. Oral Oncology. 2014;**50**(6):527-538. DOI: 10.1016/j.oraloncology.2013.12.011

[57] Stevens S, Verkuijlen S, Hariwiyanto B, Harijadi, Paramita D, Fachiroh J, et al. Noninvasive diagnosis of nasopharyngeal carcinoma: Nasopharyngeal brushings reveal high Epstein-Barr virus DNA load and carcinoma-specific viral BARF1 mRNA. International Journal of Cancer. 2006;**119**(3):608-614. DOI: 10.1002/ijc.21914

[58] Zhang G, Zong J, Lin S, Verhoeven R, Tong S, Chen Y, et al. Circulating Epstein-Barr virus microRNAs miR-BART7 and miR-BART13 as biomarkers for nasopharyngeal carcinoma diagnosis and treatment. International Journal of Cancer. 2014;**136**(5):E301-E312. DOI: 10.1002/ijc.29206

[59] Stevens S, Verkuijlen S, Hariwiyanto B, Harijadi, Fachiroh J, Paramita D, et al. Diagnostic value of measuring Epstein-Barr virus (EBV) DNA load and Carcinoma-Specific viral mRNA in relation to Anti-EBV immunoglobulin A (IgA) and IgG antibody levels in blood of nasopharyngeal carcinoma patients from Indonesia. Journal of Clinical Microbiology. 2005;**43**(7):3066-3073. DOI: 10.1128/JCM.43.7.3066-3073.2005

[60] Dales J, Beaufils N, Silvy M, Picard C, Pauly V, Pradel V, et al. Hypoxia inducible factor 1α gene (HIF-1α) splice variants: Potential prognostic biomarkers in breast cancer. BMC Medicine. 2010;**8**(1). DOI: 10.1186/1741-7015-8-44

[61] Weber D, Tille J, Combescure C, Egger J, Laouiti M, Hammad K, et al. The prognostic value of expression of HIF1α, EGFR and VEGF-A, in localized prostate cancer for intermediate- and high-risk patients treated with radiation therapy with or without androgen deprivation therapy. Radiation Oncology. 2012;**7**(1):66. DOI: 10.1186/1748-717X-7-66

[62] Valadi H, Ekström K, Bossios A, Sjöstrand M, Lee J, Lötvall J. Exosome-mediated transfer of mRNAs and microRNAs is a novel mechanism of genetic exchange between cells. Nature Cell Biology. 2007;**9**(6):654-659. DOI: 10.1038/ncb1596

[63] Hong C, Funk S, Muller L, Boyiadzis M, Whiteside T. Isolation of biologically active and morphologically intact exosomes from plasma of patients with cancer. Journal of Extracellular Vesicles. 2016;**5**:29289. DOI: 10.3402/jev.v5.29289

[64] Baranyai T, Herczeg K, Onódi Z, Voszka I, Módos K, Marton N, et al. Isolation of exosomes from blood plasma: Qualitative and quantitative comparison of ultracentrifugation and size exclusion chromatography methods. PLoS ONE. 2015;**10**(12):e0145686. DOI: 10.1371/journal.pone.0145686

[65] Tang C, Tan T, Li C, Chen Z, Ruan L, Wang G, et al. Identification of Galectin-1 as a novel biomarker in nasopharyngeal carcinoma by proteomic analysis. Oncology Reports. 2010;**24**(2):495-500. DOI: 10.3892/or_00000884

[66] Yu S, Cao H, Shen B, Feng J. Tumor-derived exosomes in cancer progression and treatment failure. Oncotarget. 2015;**6**(35):37151-37168. DOI: 10.18632/oncotarget.6022

[67] Cao Y, Yang L, Jiang W, Wang X, Liao W, Tan G, et al. Therapeutic evaluation of Epstein-Barr Virus-encoded latent membrane Protein-1 targeted DNAzyme for treating of nasopharyngeal carcinomas. Molecular Therapy. 2014;**22**(2):371-377. DOI: 10.1038/mt.2013.257

[68] Hutajulu S, Kurnianda J, Tan B, Middeldorp J. Therapeutic implications of Epstein-Barr virus infection for the treatment of nasopharyngeal carcinoma. Therapeutics and Clinical Risk Management. 2014;**10**:721-736. DOI: 10.2147/TCRM.S47434

[69] Lee H, Kim H, Kim E, Park P, Dong S, Choi T, et al. Targeted therapy for Epstein-Barr virus-associated gastric carcinoma using low-dose gemcitabine-induced lytic activation. Oncotarget. 2015;**6**(31):31018-31029. DOI: 10.18632/oncotarget.5041

[70] Stoker S, Novalić Z, Wildeman M, Huitema A, Verkuijlen S, Juwana H, et al. Epstein–Barr virus-targeted therapy in nasopharyngeal carcinoma. Journal of Cancer Research and Clinical Oncology. 2015;**141**(10):1845-1857. DOI: 10.1007/s00432-015-1969-3

[71] Chua D, Wei W, Wong M, Sham J, Nicholls J, Au G. Phase II study of gefitinib for the treatment of recurrent and metastatic nasopharyngeal carcinoma. Head & Neck. 2008;**30**(7):863-867. DOI: 10.1002/hed.20792

[72] Ma B, Hui E, King A, To K, Mo F, Leung S, et al. A phase II study of patients with metastatic or locoregionally recurrent nasopharyngeal carcinoma and evaluation of plasma Epstein–Barr virus DNA as a biomarker of efficacy. Cancer Chemotherapy and Pharmacology. 2007;**62**(1):59-64. DOI: 10.1007/s00280-007-0575-8

[73] Lee N, Zhang Q, Pfister D, Kim J, Garden A, Mechalakos J, et al. Addition of bevacizumab to standard chemoradiation for locoregionally advanced nasopharyngeal carcinoma (RTOG 0615): A phase 2 multi-institutional trial. The Lancet Oncology. 2012;**13**(2):172-180. DOI: 10.1016/S1470-2045(11):70303-70305.

[74] Elser C, Siu L, Winquist E, Agulnik M, Pond G, Chin S, et al. Phase II trial of sorafenib in patients with recurrent or metastatic squamous cell carcinoma of the head and neck or nasopharyngeal carcinoma. Journal of Clinical Oncology. 2007;**25**(24):3766-3773. DOI: 10.1200/JCO.2006.10.2871

[75] De Toro J, Herschlik L, Waldner C, Mongini C. Emerging roles of exosomes in normal and pathological conditions: New insights for diagnosis and therapeutic applications. Frontiers in Immunology. 2015;**6**:203. DOI: 10.3389/fimmu.2015.00203

[76] Marleau A, Chen C, Joyce J, Tullis R. Exosome removal as a therapeutic adjuvant in cancer. Journal of Translational Medicine. 2012;**10**(1):134. DOI: 10.1186/1479-5876-10-134

[77] Tickner J, Urquhart A, Stephenson S, Richard D, O'Byrne K. Functions and therapeutic roles of exosomes in cancer. Frontiers in Oncology. 2014;**4**:127. DOI: 10.3389/fonc.2014.00127

Section 3

Extracellular Vesicles, Microvesicles and Exosomes

Chapter 6

Mining Extracellular Vesicles for Clinically Relevant Noninvasive Diagnostic Biomarkers in Cancer

Muhammad Nawaz, Farah Fatima and
Jeremy A. Squire

Additional information is available at the end of the chapter

http://dx.doi.org/10.5772/intechopen.69406

Abstract

Extracellular vesicles (EVs) are nanosized vesicles secreted by virtually all cell types into the extracellular milieu. EVs transport bioactive molecules between cells and play multifaceted roles in cell-to-cell communications and in the pathogenesis of various human diseases including cancer. EVs are currently a focus of intensive interest, mainly because they hold a wealth of biological information in the form of differentially expressed nucleic acids and proteins, including DNA and cancer-related mutated genes, microRNAs, and a variety of transcriptional factors. Both the mutational content and any differentially expressed RNA are highly stable in patient blood or urine because they are encapsulated in EVs. This protects them against nuclease activity, pH change, temperature fluctuations, and multiple free-thaw cycles. Therefore, EVs isolated from patient fluids may serve as an ideal source of liquid biopsy for mining cancer signatures through mutation screening and genetic profiling. However, the methods for obtaining pure and intact EVs from patient samples, as well as the optimized characterization of tumor-derived EVs are still not rigorously defined for routine clinical use. High-throughput genomic or proteomic platforms may aid in the identification of novel diagnostic and prognostic biomarkers that collectively could lead to cancer monitoring and improved patient outcome.

Keywords: extracellular vesicles, exosomes, genetic profiling, biomarkers, noninvasive diagnosis, liquid biopsy, cancer

1. Introduction

Extracellular vesicles (EVs) are membrane-bounded nanosized vesicles secreted by almost every cell type studied to date. EVs carry a plethora of bioactive molecules comprising nucleic acids such as noncoding RNAs (ncRNAs), mRNA, and even DNA including both genomic and mitochondrial DNA, lipids, carbohydrates, proteins, and variety of transcriptional factors [1–3]. Based on their size, morphology, and mode of release, EVs are broadly categorized into exosomes, microvesicles, and apoptotic bodies [4]. The best characterized EVs are exosomes and microvesicles. Exosomes are produced through the endocytic pathway followed by the fusion of the multivesicular bodies (MVBs) with the plasma membrane and are released into the extracellular environment. This involves several different components of sorting machinery taking place at endosomal compartments and the MVBs (reviewed elsewhere [4]). Conversely, microvesicles are shed directly from selective microdomains of the plasma membrane and involve several components of cytoskeleton machinery.

EVs were previously considered to be platelet-derived particles and were described as cellular dust or debris until they were first recognized as specific structures termed exosomes by Johnstone et al. in 1987 [5]. Initial studies by Raposo et al. [6], Zitvogel et al. [7], and Thery et al. [8] raised the new debate that EVs are not cellular dust and highlighted the functional importance of exosomes in immunological responses. In these studies, exosomes were reported to contain major histocompatibility complex class I and class II (MHC I, MHC II) that were efficiently able to induce T-cell responses. Ratajczak and colleagues further highlighted the biological significance of secreted vesicles [9], and they were the first to report that microvesicles contain mRNA that could be transferred horizontally to target cells and subsequently translated into corresponding proteins [10, 11]. A subsequent study by Deregibus et al. reported the horizontal transfer of mRNA that was biologically associated with the activation of angiogenic program in endothelial cells [12].

The first report that exosomes contain substantial amounts of microRNA (miRNA), mRNA, and small amounts of ribosomal RNAs was documented in 2007. Valadi et al. showed that the RNAs shuttled between cells as a novel mechanism of genetic exchange between cells [13]. Following this discovery, several other studies confirmed the presence of miRNA in vesicles and showed that their transfer to neighboring cells was functional [12, 14–16]. Valadi et al. also showed that heterologous transfer of mouse EV-mRNA to recipient human mast cells is translated into corresponding mouse proteins *in vitro*, indicating that EV-mediated transfer of mRNA can be functional in recipient cells [13]. Skog et al. provided a confirmatory study showing that EV-mediated transfer of mRNA could be translated into recipient cells, which further highlights the functional role of RNA transfer [15]. Later on, Pegtel et al. showed that miRNAs secreted by EBV-infected cells were transferred to uninfected recipient cells via EVs and could potentially repress the EBV target genes [16]. Additionally, EVs from dendritic cells (DCs) could fuse with autologous target DCs and efficiently release miRNA into recipient cell cytoplasm where they repress target mRNAs of acceptor DCs [17].

1.1. Biological functions of extracellular vesicles

At the present time, the biological functions of EVs are not fully understood in comparison to well-established, paracrine-secreted factors such as cytokines and hormones. Now EVs are gaining increased attention due to their novel role in the transport of various bioactive molecules that facilitate signal transduction between cells. The secreted EVs can be taken up directly by neighboring recipient cells or they may travel through biological fluids and transport their cargo to distant organs in a paracrine manner. Considerable documented evidence emphasizes that EVs serve as mediators of cell-to-cell communication allowing the exchange of biological information between cells [18, 19]. EVs carrying diverse cargoes can move through biological fluids and thus may elicit long distance interorgan communication by dissemination of their cargo from one place to the other [20, 21]. It is possible that EVs may in fact mediate bidirectional communication and transport of regulatory molecules [22].

Due to their natural capacity in transportation and dissemination of abnormal proteins, lipids, mutated genes, and deregulated nucleic acids—EVs have been implicated in number of diseases such as neurodegenerative disease [23, 24], inflammatory and cardiovascular diseases [25, 26], and the development of cancers [15, 27–29]. The secretion and transportation of EVs from biologically active cells are likely to be context dependent, so that the signals that a particular cell receives may elicit tissue remodeling and regeneration as a response to diseases [30]. Moreover, the microbial EVs may mediate host-parasite interactions and progression of infectious diseases by disseminating virulence factors [31].

EVs derived from antigen presenting cells or cancer cells may also have a profound effect on immunomodulation, including both immune suppression and immune activation [30, 32, 33]. There is emerging role of EVs implicated in cellular differentiation, stem cell maintenance, and defining cell fates by facilitating the transmission of biological information from donor cells to recipient cells (reviewed elsewhere [22]). Such evolving roles of EVs is in part due to their abilities to mimic stem cell properties in promoting tissue's intrinsic regenerative programs and repair process within recipient cells in a paracrine manner [22]. Interestingly, the cargo of EVs is characteristic for their cell of origin, which presumably represents the disease-associated signature of their parent cells. The study of the cargo of EVs from different diseases could therefore be a rich resource for future biomarkers studies.

1.2. Extracellular vesicles as mediators of cancer initiation and metastasis

There is increased interest in how EVs may facilitate tumor progression. EVs secreted from cancer cells may carry oncogenic ncRNAs or mutated genes, which may induce aberrant gene regulation in recipient cells that induce tumor initiation [3, 14]. It is thought that EVs may educate certain recipient cells to take on a tumor-initiating phenotype. Such cells may then migrate to anatomically distinct locations leading to premetastatic colonization [28]. There are several mechanisms of tumor progression conferred by EVs including stromal remodeling, immune evasion, neovascularization, and metastasis [21, 30, 34–39]. The metastatic potential of EVs is in large part due to their ability to transmit abnormally expressed bioactive molecules such as oncoproteins, genomic and mitochondrial tumor DNA, transposon elements, and mutated genes to suitable recipient cells [14, 15, 27, 40–44].

There seems to be a strong association between EV-mediated transport of regulatory ncRNAs and the mediation of tumor initiation. EV-mediated delivery of miRNAs is thought to potentiate more diverse regulatory functions in comparison to EVs carrying other cargoes. This is mainly because EVs bearing miRNAs are capable of modulating genetic profiles of recipient cells and they may also be able to foster genomic instability [3]. It was recently shown that astrocyte-derived EVs could mediate an intercellular transfer of PTEN-targeting miRNAs to recipient primary metastatic tumor cells in order to suppress PTEN expression, and thus allowing primary tumor cells to develop metastatic potential [45]. This supports the idea that EVs are able to shuttle miRNAs between tumor cells and their metastatic progenitors. Such a reciprocal cross-talk would confer a selective advantage by facilitating coevolution of primary tumors and also favor microenvironments for adaptive metastatic outgrowth. This process could also be helped by metabolic reprogramming of tumor microenvironment. For example, recently the miRNA signatures secreted from breast cancer cells were shown to facilitate metastasis by increasing nutrient availability and reprogramming the energy metabolism of nontumor cells in a given premetastatic niche [46]. Currently, long non-coding RNAs (lncRNAs) are increasingly being reported to contribute tumor initiation and metastasis [3] and are considered as extended messages in regulating responses to chemotherapy.

2. Methods

2.1. Diversity of extracellular vesicle sources

Biological fluids and cultured cell supernatant from *in vitro* systems offer a potential source for isolation of EVs; however, EVs isolated directly from body fluids are likely to be clinically more relevant. Blood plasma is the most commonly used source for EVs collection. According to a recent survey conducted by the International Society of Extracellular Vesicles (ISEV), the plasma (47%), serum (22%), urine (14%), cerebral spinal fluid (8%), milk (5%), and miscellaneous (4%) are the relative frequencies of body fluids analyzed [47]. The choice of selecting a certain physiological fluid depends on intended downstream analysis [4].

The diverse nature of biological fluids and the individual contaminants of each fluid may represent different molecular combinations outside EVs, and may thus require different isolation methods [48]. An important bottleneck is the lack of standardized methods for collection and processing of biofluids for isolation, purification, and separation of subpopulation of EVs with removed contaminants and retained integrity of EV-cargo prerequisite for intended downstream applications. The diverse nature of biological fluids suggests that EV cargo of each fluid may represent different composition and, therefore, a spectrum of methods will need to be considered to define contaminants of each fluid in order to obtain pure EVs.

2.1.1. Available techniques for EV isolation

There are a variety of methods available and more are being developed, some of them are poorly standardized. These include ultrafiltration, density gradient centrifugation, size exclusion chromatography and affinity isolation, polymeric precipitation, and the microfluidic devices [48]. Each method has variable isolation efficiencies when applied to different samples, such as blood plasma, milk, urine, and cell culture media.

A comparison of several conventional as well as high-throughput technologies for the isolation and characterization of different samples has been recently undertaken with a focus on their advantages and disadvantages [4]. Recently, the ISEV has made a critical analysis of various techniques implemented for isolation of EVs and they have made potential recommendations [48, 49]. Differential ultracentrifugation remains the most widely used primary isolation method, comparable to several other techniques, and is suitable for large-volume isolations. However, for the isolation of EVs from low volume samples, it was found that size exclusion chromatography is now a more widely used technique, which allows separation of EV from the bulk of soluble proteins. In this method, the separation is purely based on particle size, therefore contaminating particles in the EV size range such as lipoprotein complexes may be coisolated [48, 50]. When the intent is to capture a selective class of EVs, immunoaffinity capture offers an alternative method with a much higher selective specificity. The method can yield pure EV subpopulations, but is highly influenced by both the choice of affinity reagent and the ligand density on different EV types [48].

Other methods include microfluidic devices, filtration, and various commercially available kits. The commercial kits often make the use of volume-excluding polymers, such as polyethylene glycol (PEG), which enables rapid EV isolation from culture media or from body fluids. However, such polymers may also coprecipitate protein complexes that can contaminate EV isolates. Therefore, the ISEV has recommended using two different EV isolation techniques that are based on distinct principles of separation and each will thus enrich for different subpopulations of vesicles. Since each method potentially coisolates the contaminants, such as protein complexes and lipoproteins to different degrees, the ISEV proposes that a combination of techniques be applied, such as density gradient centrifugation followed by size exclusion or immunoaffinity capture [48].

The method of choice should take into account several factors: sample type, volume, yield, integrity, purity of EVs required for specific downstream analysis, as well as the available instrumentation and processing time [4]. The chosen method will be influenced by whether the sample is derived from cell-culture media or from body-fluids and whether the intended analysis is proteomic or genomic. Therefore, the choice of different isolation methods for EVs will impact the amount, type, and purity of EVs recovered and will guide the type of downstream analysis of EVs that is the most practical.

2.2. Characterization of EVs and available analytical technologies

After the isolation procedures, one needs to characterize EVs for their size determination, detection of common EVs marker, morphology, and concentration (quantification), for which there is a variety of techniques available [4, 51, 52]. Characterization of EVs currently presents various challenges, mainly due to their small size, the complexity of the EV cargo, and the physical parameters of available instruments for measuring nanosized EVs. Given the fact that EVs are isolated from a variety of different sources with highly variable composition (as stated above), it is difficult to provide general recommendations for EV isolation and characterization. The sample type, sample volume, and the choice of downstream application all will be an influence on the characterization instruments employed.

The mean size and overall size distribution of individual subpopulations of EVs, as well as their relative abundance, can be determined by nanotracking analysis (NTA), Zetaview [53–60], and tunable resistive pulse sensing (qNANO) [61]. Electron microscopy is used to assess the submicron phenotype of EVs [51, 59, 62–64], whereas flow cytometry is used for enumerating, phenotyping, and sorting of EVs based on their size distribution [65, 66]. Western blotting is implemented when the aim is to detect EV-markers such as CD63, CD81, and CD9. A recent survey conducted by ISEV has mentioned that the three most widely used techniques for EVs characterization are Western blotting (74%), single-particle tracking (SPT, 72%), and electron microscopy (60%) [47].

Hitherto, the flow cytometry remains a popular tool for measuring EVs [65, 66]; however, fundamental principles and limitations of the instrument need to be considered [67]. EVs isolated by ultracentrifugation may cause aggregation of EVs thus rendering subsequent difficulties for flow cytometric analysis or single particle tracking analysis [47], whereas, those isolated using size exclusion kits may lead to subsequent difficulties for downstream EV analysis by Western blotting. Recently, tunable resistive pulse sensing has been used to precisely determine the concentration of EVs. Further validations are required to show that this promising new method is reproducible and widely applicable for characterizing EVs [61].

The characterization of heterogeneous subpopulations of EVs into their component parts remains an unresolved issue. This problem of EV subclassification arises because almost all subtypes, including exosomes and microvesicles, share same/common EV detection markers such as CD63, CD81, and CD9 [48, 52]. Recent papers claim successful subclassification EVs based on general surface protein profiling (proteomics) [57, 68] or on RNA content profiling (RNAomics) of individual EV populations [69–73]. New advances in both EV isolation techniques and detailed optimization and standardization of existing techniques or protocols will facilitate progress toward more precise and reliable EV characterization. These crucial steps will greatly influence the identification of specific biomarkers in EV subpopulations.

2.2.1. Characterization and profiling of nucleic acid content from EVs: potential issues

Prior to profiling of RNA content from EVs, it is important to assess the quality of RNA. There are predominantly two populations of secreted extracellular RNA (exRNA) either in association with RNA-binding proteins, or as a part of lipoprotein complexes, or alternatively vesicle bound RNAs. It is thought that such protein complexes might be coprecipitated and coisolated along with EVs during ultra-centrifugation. Therefore, the methods that remove contaminating proteins from EV aggregates are highly required.

The occurrence of extracellular RNA (exRNA) either inside secreted EVs or outside EVs (i.e., non-EV exRNA) is a controversial subject at the present time, as there are discrepancies in the results shown by different laboratories [74–78]. In order to discriminate RNA encapsulated within/or on the surface of EVs from those non-EV bound exRNA, it is critical to digest isolated RNA fractions with RNase and proteinase to disrupt the ribonucleoproteins and any RNA exterior to vesicles [48]. This procedure will deplete non-EV exRNA leaving behind EV-encapsulated RNA.

A potential issue in studies using *in vitro* methods is the fetal bovine serum (FBS) that is used for cell cultures. FBS already contains various bovine RNA species that are retained even after extended period of ultracentrifugation during the preparations of the vesicle-depleted FBS [79]. This raises the possibility that the RNA being analyzed might not be exclusively from human vesicles and subsequent qPCR or sequencing analysis may contain artifactual bovine nucleic acids derived from nonvesicular bound RNA, which may bias results [80].

An additional issue related to expression analysis, and sequencing library preparations from EV-RNA; is the low input sample material. Particularly this refers to small sample source e.g., less EV-RNA from low volume of patient blood or the usage of low recovery protocol). Low input material may suffer biases not only when the library is prepared but also during the EV-RNA ligation step. Measuring the quantity and integrity of EV-associated RNA is challenging due to limited amount of RNA available and the lack of reference standards, such as those established for cellular mRNA. Recently, the ISEV has addressed these issues and have made recommendations for the assessment and analysis of the nature of EV-associated RNAs [48]. Detection of the levels of certain transcripts by highly sensitive RT-qPCR may be used as a proxy for total RNA quantification in samples containing a low abundance of RNA.

Sensitive techniques, such as Agilent Bioanalyzer pico chip and the Quant-iT RiboGreen RNA Assay, have been proven to be more suitable methods for the quantification EV-RNA than that of Nanodrop method. Most of the techniques (with the exception of the Qubit RNA HS Assay) are thought to be sensitive to DNA contamination. Therefore, ISEV recommends pretreatment of samples with DNase for accurate RNA quantitation [48]. Due to the enrichment of small RNA species in EVs, the main focus of recent studies is the assessment of miRNAs and other small ncRNAs. Such studies take into consideration subsequent expression analyses and deep sequencing experiments. ISEV has provided recommendations on the different steps of EV-RNA analysis, such as RT-qPCR analysis, selection of reference genes, deep sequencing, library preparation, biases issues, data normalization, and bioinformatics analysis.

3. Genetic profiling of EVs from cancer-derived biofluids: a stable source of noninvasive diagnosis

In the absence of early symptoms, most cancers are diagnosed at an advanced stage, by which time patients have poor outcomes and tumors have often metastasized. Pathological evaluations and resulting treatment approaches are often determined based on biopsy material. The detection of biomarkers from body fluids may offer significant advantage over the use of tissue markers, because biopsies are invasive procedures and are associated with bleeding and risk of infections. Moreover, biopsies are often difficult to perform for organs that lie deep within the body and may suffer from sample bias [81].

There is an intensive interest in mining biological fluids as a noninvasive source of biomarkers detection. For example, elevated prostate-specific antigen (PSA) levels in plasma are routinely used for the early detection and monitoring of prostate cancer. However, since the blood levels of this assay vary widely, PSA testing often fails to detect a new cancer or to accurately predict disease stage. Novel more precise blood and urine biomarkers are needed at both diagnosis and during the disease progression of prostate cancer [82]. The expression levels of miRNAs in prostate cancer show considerable promise as potential biomarkers with clinical applications. Since the miRNA content of EVs reflects the miRNA expression profile of the cells they originated from, there has been considerable interest in mining miRNAs from EVs in prostate cancer. One good example is miR-16, which has increased expression in plasma from metastatic prostate cancer patients, but has reduced levels of expression in both primary and metastatic prostate cancer tissue RNA samples [83]. In contrast, miR-21 was found to be elevated in the early disease, but not in advanced prostate cancer [84]. One of the most powerful applications could be early detecting of prostate cancer in patients' urine. An agglutination methods were used recently to isolate miRNAs from prostate cancer urine, which showed that upregulation of miR-574-3p, miR-141-5p, and miR-21-5p was associated with disease [85].

Since deregulated miRNA expression is an early event in tumorigenesis, measuring circulating miRNA levels could be potentially useful for early cancer detection, and may contribute to greatly measure the success of treatment or evaluate the therapeutic response.

4. Mining extracellular vesicles for cancer diagnosis

Proteins and nucleic acids encapsulated within EVs circulating in body fluids are thought to be more stable against proteases and nucleases that are naturally present in body fluids. The protection of nucleic acids in EVs provides a great advantage of storage conditions as well as handling at adverse physical conditions such as fluctuations in temperature and changes in pH, multiple freeze, and thaw cycles, and thus could be an appealing source for biomarker development [4]. Moreover, circulating EVs from cancer patients have been found to express signatures that are significantly distinct from profiles of benign disease or normal controls [86–88].

Interestingly, tumor cells release EVs containing tumor-specific content that could be easily isolated from various body fluids such as blood plasma, serum, and urine. In this regard, EV-assisted liquid biopsies offer an inherent advantage, mainly because samples could be collected longitudinally with great ease and in large quantities (i.e., sample reproducibility). EVs release is an active process and tumor cells can shed plenty of EVs per milliliter of plasma [89]. EVs released into body fluids containing differentially or aberrantly expressed miRNAs often retain the characteristics of the tumors from which they originated [15, 87, 90]. Interestingly, it has been proposed that the cellular origin of EVs from certain cancer types or cell types could be used to determine the likely identity of an unknown disease [91]. This may assist the assessment of EVs in a body fluid from new cancer patients when there is uncertainty about the type of tumor. Consequently, EVs from biological fluids could be subjected to large-scale screening of tumor-specific markers [33, 40, 89, 92–95].

The comprehensive detection of diverse EV components, in particular the profiling of EV-linked ncRNAs including short ncRNAs such as miRNAs, as well as lncRNAs from peripheral blood or urine of cancer patients, may be a source of predictive cancer signatures for early diagnosis of specific cancer types. There is already evidence for using exRNA including vesicle bound and nonvesicle bound exRNA comprising circulatory miRNAs and lncRNAs from human body fluids for determining diagnostic and prognostic value of RNA signatures related to cancer [3]. In this context, the presence of ncRNA in EVs may serve an additional platform for biomarker discovery. The global profiling of EV-encapsulated RNAs with mutation characterization and/or without mutation characterization [33] could serve as a potential source for cancer detection. This could allow clinicians to perform patient stratification (companion diagnostics), screening, monitoring treatment response, and detection of minimal residual disease after surgery/recurrence [89].

miRNA profiling from EpCAM-positive EVs from serum of ovarian cancer patients demonstrated that EV-derived miRNA signatures from advanced stage patients are significantly distinct from those at benign stage, providing a possible biomarker signature to distinguish early stage cancer from advanced disease [87]. Expression of candidate cell-free urine miRNAs in ovarian cancer and endometrial cancer patients has demonstrated their prospective use as biomarkers [96]. However, in order to confirm the diagnostic potential of urine miRNAs in gynecological cancers, it requires large number of clinical samples and large-scale expression profiling studies. Additionally, mining EVs from urine samples of cancer patients may help early diagnosis. In this context, the most often studied cancer for mining urinary EVs is the prostate cancer [97–107].

In addition to their utility in diagnostic platforms, the EV-associated cargo from serum/plasma may also serve as bona fide signatures of disease prognosis, tumor recurrence, and overall survival. This refers to prognostic implications against chemotherapies as well as radiotherapies related to several cancer types. Therefore, the ncRNA signatures from EV sources may have clinical implications. However, it is critical to compare and standardize results of global investigations regarding EV-associated circulating ncRNAs as well as the recommendations for preanalytic considerations in biomarker discovery.

Although, the biological consequences of the discriminatory distribution of miRNAs in EVs are not fully known, it is possible that measuring the concentration of miRNAs from biological fluids (i.e., blood, urine serous, and ascites) and making corresponding comparisons could allow biomarker identification. Interestingly, the miR-21, one the global tumor marker, is found in EVs from serum and plasma of various cancer types and may serve as an independent marker of tumor diagnosis and prognosis [33, 108–110]. Presumably, the global profiling or selective screening of EV-RNAs against mutations may predict tumor-specific signature, whereas the enrichment on ncRNAs within tumor cell-derived EVs could offer a promising platform for developing disease biomarkers.

Another area of interest for EVs in cancer is their potential to restore gene activity that has been lost. PTEN is frequently deleted in prostate cancer and associated with aggressive disease [111]. Using an *in vitro* system it was shown that through EVs the PTEN can be transferred back into cells that have lost PTEN expression [82]. Interestingly, the transferred PTEN was competent to confer tumor suppression, suggesting that exosomal PTEN may in the future be able compensate for PTEN loss in PTEN-deficient prostate cancers. Initially, it was shown that cancer cells release PTEN via EVs and could be transferred to other cells through EVs [112]. In cells that exhibit a reduction of PTEN expression or complete loss of PTEN expression, the tumor-suppression activity was restored via EV-mediated transfer of PTEN to acceptor cells. Interestingly, PTEN could be detected from EVs that circulate in the blood of prostate cancer patients. Conversely, the normal subjects have no PTEN expression in their blood EVs. Moreover, the prostate-specific antigen (PSA) was also detected in EVs derived from prostate cancer patients. These data suggest that EV-associated PTEN can not only compensate for PTEN loss in PTEN deficient cells, but also may have diagnostic value for prostate cancer [112]. The workflow to mining EVs for nucleic acid analysis and proteomic profiling is given in **Figure 1**.

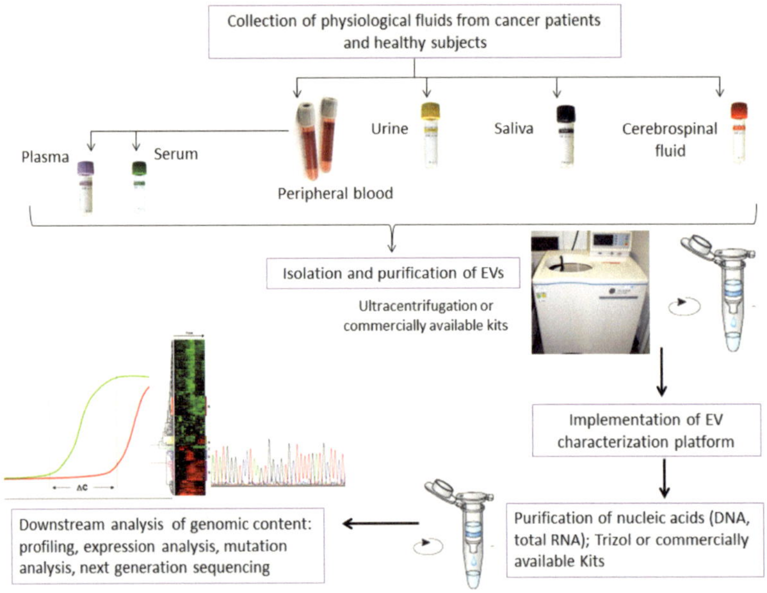

Figure 1. A flow sheet of extracellular vesicle (EV) isolation and analysis: for utilizing EVs as biomarkers, the physiological fluids from cancer patients and healthy subjects are collected, and EVs are isolated from various fluids. EVs from each source need to be characterized and EV-RNA is isolated for downstream analysis in order to identify genetic aberrations or profiling of genomic content.

5. Conclusion

There is still a long way to go to fully understand EV content in the context of cancer as a systemic disease. It will be necessary to establish a link between tumor occurrence, progression, treatment response, and corresponding changes in EV content. Since biopsies are associated with potential risk factors such as surgical resection and associated toxicity, alternative methods will be required for early diagnosis. The longitudinal collection of EVs from patient body fluids may offer untapped source for liquid biopsy. As such, the EVs cargo itself may represent an attractive source of multiple candidate biomarkers that could provide clinically useful information for cancer management. The ease with which EVs can be collected and purified from body fluids suggests that biomarkers present in their cargo could eventually be part of personalized cancer care, possibly replacing more invasive biopsies.

The detection of candidate molecules anchored to circulating EVs, may thus allow cancers to be identified from several drops of a patient blood, and may serve as highly sensitive screening tools [113]. Therefore, EVs are ideal source of screening intact molecular signatures of tumor origin. EV-associated ncRNAs including miRNAs as well as lncRNAs are currently the most frequently exploited biomarkers for cancer diagnosis [3]. Identification of aberrantly expressed RNA molecules, mutated genes, or proteins in EVs from body fluids of cancer patients can be subjected to next-generation genomics and proteomics approaches that may aid in the identification of diagnostic and prognostic biomarkers.

To be able to use EVs as liquid biopsies, a comprehensive inventory of their constituents such as proteins, DNA, RNA, and metabolites, followed by the validation of distinct candidates in the frame of a multicenter clinical study is required (see workflow for biomarker development [4]). However, the noninvasive detection technologies should be accurate, fast, and potentially inexpensive.

It has been argued that the development of high-throughput approaches and robust capture platforms will warrant the implications of EVs in routine biomarker development, and therapeutic implications with a proposed workflow sheet to be applied for US Food and Drug Administration (FDA) approval [4]. What needs to be considered as a priority is the standardization of scientific reporting. At present, differences in reporting approaches could make it difficult to compare and standardize the potential therapeutic effects of EVs. Such inconsistencies may limit the likelihood of translating EVs into human clinical trials. Efforts are being made to ensure transparent reporting of EV findings in order to facilitate interpretation and replication of experiments [114]. This will help to put experimental guidelines into practice. Since there is intensive interest in the field both in basic research as well as therapeutic point of view, it is anticipated that in the next decade, EVs arena will see significant advances in clinical pipelines [32].

Acknowledgements

This work was supported by FAPESP (Sao Paulo Research Foundation, Proc. No. 2015/09111-5 to J. A. Squire. M. Nawaz acknowledges FAPESP (Sao Paulo Research Foundation, Proc. No. 12/24574-3) and CAPES (Coordination for the Improvement of Higher Education Personnel, Proc. No. BEX 7057/15-6). F. Fatima acknowledges CAPES (Coordination for the Improvement of Higher Education Personnel, Proc. No. BEX 6332/15-3) Brazil.

Conflict of interest

The authors of this chapter declare that there is no conflict of interest.

Author details

Muhammad Nawaz[1,2]*, Farah Fatima[1,2] and Jeremy A. Squire[1,3]

*Address all correspondence to: nawazm.edu@gmail.com

1 Department of Pathology and Forensic Medicine, Ribeirão Preto Medical School, University of São Paulo, Ribeirão Preto, Brazil

2 Department of Rheumatology and Inflammation Research, Sahlgrenska Academy, University of Gothenburg, Gothenburg, Sweden

3 Department of Pathology and Molecular Medicine, Queen's University, Kingston, Canada

References

[1] Keerthikumar S, et al. ExoCarta: A web-based compendium of exosomal cargo. Journal of Molecular Biology. 2016;**428**(4):688-692

[2] Kim DK. et al. EVpedia: A community web portal for extracellular vesicles research. Bioinformatics. 2015;**31**(6):933-939

[3] Fatima F, Nawaz M. Vesiculated long non-coding RNAs: Offshore packages deciphering Trans-Regulation between cells, cancer progression and resistance to therapies. Non-Coding RNA. 2017;**3**(1):10

[4] Nawaz M, et al. The emerging role of extracellular vesicles as biomarkers for urogenital cancers. Nature Reviews Urology 2014;**11**(12):688-701

[5] Johnstone RM, et al. Vesicle formation during reticulocyte maturation. Association of plasma membrane activities with released vesicles (exosomes). Journal of Biological Chemistry 1987;**262**(19):9412-9420

[6] Raposo G, et al. B lymphocytes secrete antigen-presenting vesicles. Journal of Experimental Medicine. 1996;**183**(3):1161-1172

[7] Zitvogel L, et al. Eradication of established murine tumors using a novel cell-free vaccine: Dendritic cell-derived exosomes. Nature Medicine. 1998;**4**(5):594-600

[8] Thery C, et al. Molecular characterization of dendritic cell-derived exosomes. Selective accumulation of the heat shock protein hsc73. Journal of Cell Biology. 1999;**147**(3):599-610

[9] Ratajczak J, et al. Biological significance of the different erythropoietic factors secreted by normal human early erythroid cells. Leukemia and Lymphoma. 2003;**44**(5):767-774

[10] Ratajczak J, et al. Embryonic stem cell-derived microvesicles reprogram hematopoietic progenitors: Evidence for horizontal transfer of mRNA and protein delivery. Leukemia. 2006;**20**(5):847-856

[11] Baj-Krzyworzeka M, et al. Tumour-derived microvesicles carry several surface determinants and mRNA of tumour cells and transfer some of these determinants to monocytes. Cancer Immunology, Immunotherapy. 2006;**55**(7):808-818

[12] Deregibus MC, et al. Endothelial progenitor cell derived microvesicles activate an angiogenic program in endothelial cells by a horizontal transfer of mRNA. Blood. 2007;**110**(7):2440-2448

[13] Valadi H, et al. Exosome-mediated transfer of mRNAs and microRNAs is a novel mechanism of genetic exchange between cells. Nature Cell Biology. 2007;**9**(6):654-659

[14] Al-Nedawi K, et al. Intercellular transfer of the oncogenic receptor EGFRvIII by microvesicles derived from tumour cells. Nature Cell Biology. 2008;**10**(5):619-624

[15] Skog J, et al. Glioblastoma microvesicles transport RNA and proteins that promote tumour growth and provide diagnostic biomarkers. Nature Cell Biology. 2008;**10**(12):1470-1476

[16] Pegtel DM, et al. Functional delivery of viral miRNAs via exosomes. Proceedings of the National Academy of Sciences. 2010;**107**(14):6328-6333

[17] Montecalvo A, et al. Mechanism of transfer of functional microRNAs between mouse dendritic cells via exosomes. Blood. 2012;**119**(3):756-766

[18] Mathivanan S, Ji H, Simpson RJ. Exosomes: Extracellular organelles important in intercellular communication. Journal of Proteomics. 2010;**73**(10):1907-1920

[19] Raposo G, Stoorvogel W. Extracellular vesicles: Exosomes, microvesicles, and friends. Journal of Cell Biology. 2013;**200**(4):373-383

[20] Thomou T, et al. Adipose-derived circulating miRNAs regulate gene expression in other tissues. Nature. 2017;**542**(7642):450-455

[21] Hoshino, A., et al. Tumour exosome integrins determine organotropic metastasis. Nature. 2015;**527**(7578):pp. 329-335.

[22] Nawaz M, et al. Extracellular vesicles: Evolving factors in stem cell biology. Stem Cells International. 2016;**2016**:1073140

[23] Rajendran L, et al. Alzheimer's disease beta-amyloid peptides are released in association with exosomes. Proceedings of the National Academy of Sciences. 2006;**103**(30): 11172-11177

[24] Vella LJ, et al. The role of exosomes in the processing of proteins associated with neurodegenerative diseases. European Biophysics Journal. 2008;**37**(3):323-332

[25] Buzas EI, et al. Emerging role of extracellular vesicles in inflammatory diseases. Nature Reviews Rheumatology. 2014;**10**(6):356-364

[26] Osteikoetxea X, et al. Extracellular vesicles in cardiovascular disease: Are they Jedi or Sith?. Journal of Physiology. 2016;**594**(11):2881-2894

[27] Al-Nedawi K, et al. Endothelial expression of autocrine VEGF upon the uptake of tumor-derived microvesicles containing oncogenic EGFR. Proceedings of the National Academy of Sciences. 2009;**106**(10):3794-3799

[28] Peinado H, et al. Melanoma exosomes educate bone marrow progenitor cells toward a pro-metastatic phenotype through MET. Nature Medicine. 2012;**18**(6):883-891

[29] Nawaz M, et al. Microvesicles in gliomas and medulloblastomas: An overview. Journal of Cancer Therapy. 2014;**5**(2):10

[30] Fatima F, Nawaz M. Stem cell-derived exosomes: Roles in stromal remodeling, tumor progression, and cancer immunotherapy. Chinese Journal of Cancer. 2015;**34**(12):541-553

[31] Schwab A, et al. Extracellular vesicles from infected cells: Potential for direct pathogenesis. Frontiers in Microbiology. 2015;**6**:1132

[32] Fatima F, Nawaz M. Nexus between extracellular vesicles, immunomodulation and tissue remodeling: For good or for bad? Annals of Translational Medicine. 2017;**5**(6):139

[33] Nawaz M, et al. Extracellular vesicles in ovarian cancer: Applications to tumor biology, immunotherapy and biomarker discovery. Expert Review of Proteomics. 2016; **13**(4):395-409

[34] Janowska-Wieczorek A, et al. Microvesicles derived from activated platelets induce metastasis and angiogenesis in lung cancer. International Journal of Cancer. 2005; **113**(5):752-760

[35] Janowska-Wieczorek A, et al. Enhancing effect of platelet-derived microvesicles on the invasive potential of breast cancer cells. Transfusion. 2006;**46**(7):1199-1209

[36] Costa-Silva B, et al. Pancreatic cancer exosomes initiate pre-metastatic niche formation in the liver. Nature Cell Biology. 2015;**17**(6):816-826

[37] Lima LG, et al. Tumor-derived microvesicles modulate the establishment of metastatic melanoma in a phosphatidylserine-dependent manner. Cancer Letters. 2009;**283**(2): 168-175

[38] Greening DW, et al. Emerging roles of exosomes during epithelial-mesenchymal transition and cancer progression. Seminars in Cell and Developmental Biology. 2015;**40**:60-71

[39] Taverna S, et al. Exosomal shuttling of miR-126 in endothelial cells modulates adhesive and migratory abilities of chronic myelogenous leukemia cells. Molecular Cancer. 2014;**13**:169

[40] Balaj L, et al. Tumour microvesicles contain retrotransposon elements and amplified oncogene sequences. Nature Communications. 2011;**2**:180

[41] Guescini M, et al. Astrocytes and Glioblastoma cells release exosomes carrying mtDNA. Journal of Neural Transmission (Vienna). 2010;**117**(1):1-4

[42] Greening DW, et al. Secreted primary human malignant mesothelioma exosome signature reflects oncogenic cargo. Science Report. 2016;**6**:32643

[43] Di Vizio D, et al. Large oncosomes in human prostate cancer tissues and in the circulation of mice with metastatic disease. American Journal of Pathology. 2012;**181**(5):1573-1584

[44] Morello M, et al. Large oncosomes mediate intercellular transfer of functional microRNA. Cell Cycle. 2013;**12**(22):3526-3536

[45] Zhang L, et al. Microenvironment-induced PTEN loss by exosomal microRNA primes brain metastasis outgrowth. Nature. 2015;**527**(7576):100-104

[46] Fong MY, et al. Breast-cancer-secreted miR-122 reprograms glucose metabolism in premetastatic niche to promote metastasis. Nature Cell Biology. 2015;**17**(2):183-194

[47] Gardiner C, et al. Techniques used for the isolation and characterization of extracellular vesicles: Results of a worldwide survey. Journal of Extracellular Vesicles. 2016;**5**:32945

[48] Mateescu B, et al. Obstacles and opportunities in the functional analysis of extracellular vesicle RNA – an ISEV position paper. Journal of Extracellular Vesicles. 2017;**6**(1):1286095

[49] Witwer KW, et al. Standardization of sample collection, isolation and analysis methods in extracellular vesicle research. Journal of Extracellular Vesicles. 2013;**2**

[50] Sodar BW, et al. Low-density lipoprotein mimics blood plasma-derived exosomes and microvesicles during isolation and detection. Science Report. 2016;**6**:24316

[51] Rupert DL, et al. Methods for the physical characterization and quantification of extracellular vesicles in biological samples. Biochimica et Biophysica Acta. 2017;**1861**(1 Pt A):3164-3179

[52] Maas SL, et al. Possibilities and limitations of current technologies for quantification of biological extracellular vesicles and synthetic mimics. Journal of Controlled Release. 2015;**200**:87-96

[53] Baldwin S, et al. Analyzing the miRNA content of extracellular vesicles by fluorescence nanoparticle tracking. Nanomedicine. 2016;**13**(2):765-770

[54] Dragovic RA, et al. Sizing and phenotyping of cellular vesicles using Nanoparticle Tracking Analysis. Nanomedicine. 2011;**7**(6):780-788

[55] Gardiner C, et al. Extracellular vesicle sizing and enumeration by nanoparticle tracking analysis. Journal of Extracellular Vesicles. 2013;**2**

[56] Pachler K, et al. A Good Manufacturing Practice-grade standard protocol for exclusively human mesenchymal stromal cell-derived extracellular vesicles. Cytotherapy. 2017;**19**(4):458-472

[57] Kibria G, et al. A rapid, automated surface protein profiling of single circulating exosomes in human blood. Science Report. 2016;**6**:36502

[58] Nardi Fda S, et al. High levels of circulating extracellular vesicles with altered expression and function during pregnancy. Immunobiology. 2016;**221**(7):753-760

[59] van der Pol E, et al. Particle size distribution of exosomes and microvesicles determined by transmission electron microscopy, flow cytometry, nanoparticle tracking analysis, and resistive pulse sensing. Journal of Thrombosis and Haemostasis. 2014;**12**(7):1182-1192

[60] Dragovic RA, et al. Isolation of syncytiotrophoblast microvesicles and exosomes and their characterisation by multicolour flow cytometry and fluorescence nanoparticle tracking analysis. Methods. 2015;**87**:64-74

[61] Vogel R, et al. A standardized method to determine the concentration of extracellular vesicles using tunable resistive pulse sensing. Journal of Extracellular Vesicles. 2016;**5**:31242

[62] Fertig ET, Gherghiceanu M, Popescu LM. Extracellular vesicles release by cardiac telocytes: Electron microscopy and electron tomography. Journal of Cellular and Molecular Medicine. 2014;**18**(10):1938-1943

[63] Brisson AR, et al. Extracellular vesicles from activated platelets: A semiquantitative cryo-electron microscopy and immuno-gold labeling study. Platelets. 2017;**28**(3):263-271

[64] Hoog JL, Lotvall J. Diversity of extracellular vesicles in human ejaculates revealed by cryo-electron microscopy. Journal of Extracellular Vesicles. 2015;**4**:28680

[65] Groot Kormelink T, et al. Prerequisites for the analysis and sorting of extracellular vesicle subpopulations by high-resolution flow cytometry. Cytometry A. 2016;**89**(2):135-147

[66] van der Vlist EJ, et al. Fluorescent labeling of nano-sized vesicles released by cells and subsequent quantitative and qualitative analysis by high-resolution flow cytometry. Nature Protocols. 2012;**7**(7):1311-1326

[67] Nolan JP. Flow cytometry of extracellular vesicles: Potential, pitfalls, and prospects. Current Protocols in Cytometry. 2015;**73**:13 14 1-16

[68] Kowal J, et al. Proteomic comparison defines novel markers to characterize heterogeneous populations of extracellular vesicle subtypes. Proceedings of the National Academy of Sciences. 2016;**113**(8):E968-E977

[69] Lasser C, et al. Two distinct extracellular RNA signatures released by a single cell type identified by microarray and next-generation sequencing. RNA Biology. 2017;**14**(1):58-72

[70] Lunavat TR, et al. Small RNA deep sequencing discriminates subsets of extracellular vesicles released by melanoma cells--Evidence of unique microRNA cargos. RNA Biology. 2015;**12**(8):810-823

[71] Crescitelli R, et al. Distinct RNA profiles in subpopulations of extracellular vesicles: Apoptotic bodies, microvesicles and exosomes. Journal of Extracellular Vesicles. 2013;**2**

[72] Conley A, et al. High-throughput sequencing of two populations of extracellular vesicles provides an mRNA signature that can be detected in the circulation of breast cancer patients. RNA Biology. 2016;**14**(3):305-316

[73] Huang X, et al. Characterization of human plasma-derived exosomal RNAs by deep sequencing. BMC Genomics. 2013;**14**:319

[74] Arroyo JD, et al. Argonaute2 complexes carry a population of circulating microRNAs independent of vesicles in human plasma. Proceedings of the National Academy of Sciences. 2011;**108**(12):5003-5008

[75] Turchinovich A, et al. Characterization of extracellular circulating microRNA. Nucleic Acids Research. 2011;**39**(16):7223-7233

[76] Gourzones C, et al. Consistent high concentration of the viral microRNA BART17 in plasma samples from nasopharyngeal carcinoma patients--evidence of non-exosomal transport. Virology Journal. 2013;**10**:119

[77] Chevillet JR, et al. Quantitative and stoichiometric analysis of the microRNA content of exosomes. Proceedings of the National Academy of Sciences 2014;**111**(41):14888-14893

[78] Patton JG, et al. Biogenesis, delivery, and function of extracellular RNA. Journal of Extracellular Vesicles. 2015;**4**:27494

[79] Wei Z, et al. Fetal bovine serum RNA interferes with the cell culture derived extracellular RNA. Science Report. 2016;**6**:31175

[80] Tosar JP, et al. Ribonucleic artefacts: Are some extracellular RNA discoveries driven by cell culture medium components? Journal of Extracellular Vesicles. 2017;**6**(1):1272832

[81] Bedard PL, et al. Tumour heterogeneity in the clinic. Nature. 2013;**501**(7467):355-364

[82] Valentino A, et al. Exosomal microRNAs in liquid biopsies: Future biomarkers for prostate cancer. Clinical and Translational Oncology. 2017;**19**(6):651-657

[83] Bonci D, et al. The miR-15a-miR-16-1 cluster controls prostate cancer by targeting multiple oncogenic activities. Nature Medicine. 2008;**14**(11):1271-127

[84] Hizir MS, et al. Simultaneous detection of circulating oncomiRs from body fluids for prostate cancer staging using nanographene oxide. ACS Applied Materials & Interfaces. 2014;**6**(17):14772-14778

[85] Samsonov R, et al. Lectin-induced agglutination method of urinary exosomes isolation followed by mi-RNA analysis: Application for prostate cancer diagnostic. Prostate. 2016;**76**(1):68-79

[86] Graves LE, et al. Proinvasive properties of ovarian cancer ascites-derived membrane vesicles. Cancer Research. 2004;**64**(19):7045-7049

[87] Taylor DD, Gercel-Taylor C. MicroRNA signatures of tumor-derived exosomes as diagnostic biomarkers of ovarian cancer. Gynecologic Oncology. 2008;**110**(1):13-21

[88] Rank A, et al. Circulating microparticles in patients with benign and malignant ovarian tumors. Anticancer Research. 2012;**32**(5):2009-2014

[89] Brock G, Castellanos-Rizaldos E, Hu L, Coticchia C, Skog J. Liquid biopsy for cancer screening, patient stratification and monitoring. Translational Cancer Research. 2015;**4**(3):280-290

[90] Kuhlmann JD, et al. microRNA and the pathogenesis of ovarian cancer--a new horizon for molecular diagnostics and treatment? Clinical Chemistry and Laboratory Medicine. 2012;**50**(4):601-615

[91] Larssen P, et al. Tracing cellular origin of human exosomes using multiplex proximity extension assay. Molecular & Cellular Proteomics. 2017;**16**(3):502-511

[92] Kahlert C, et al. Identification of double-stranded genomic DNA spanning all chromosomes with mutated KRAS and p53 DNA in the serum exosomes of patients with pancreatic cancer. Journal of Biological Chemistry. 2014;**289**(7):3869-3875

[93] Royo F, et al. Comparative miRNA analysis of urine extracellular vesicles isolated through five different methods. Cancers (Basel). 2016;**8**(12)

[94] Krafft C, et al. A specific spectral signature of serum and plasma-derived extracellular vesicles for cancer screening. Nanomedicine. 2017;**13**(3):835-841

[95] Cappello F, et al. Exosome levels in human body fluids: A tumor marker by themselves? European Journal of Pharmaceutical Sciences. 2017;**96**:93-98

[96] Zavesky L, et al. Evaluation of Cell-Free urine microRNAs expression for the use in diagnosis of ovarian and endometrial cancers. A pilot study. Pathology and Oncology Research. 2015;**21**(4):1027-1035

[97] Mitchell PJ, et al. Can urinary exosomes act as treatment response markers in prostate cancer? Journal of Translational Medicine. 2009;**7**:4

[98] Nilsson J, et al. Prostate cancer-derived urine exosomes: A novel approach to biomarkers for prostate cancer. British Journal of Cancer. 2009;**100**(10):1603-1607

[99] Motamedinia P, et al. Urine exosomes for Non-Invasive assessment of gene expression and mutations of prostate cancer. PLoS One. 2016;**11**(5):e0154507

[100] Royo F, et al. Transcriptomic profiling of urine extracellular vesicles reveals alterations of CDH3 in prostate cancer. Oncotarget. 2016;**7**(6):6835-6846

[101] Hendriks RJ, et al. Comparative analysis of prostate cancer specific biomarkers PCA3 and ERG in whole urine, urinary sediments and exosomes. Clinical Chemistry and Laboratory Medicine. 2016;**54**(3):483-492

[102] Huang X, et al. Exosomal miR-1290 and miR-375 as prognostic markers in castration-resistant prostate cancer. European Journal of Urology. 2015;**67**(1):33-41

[103] Ahadi A, et al. Long non-coding RNAs harboring miRNA seed regions are enriched in prostate cancer exosomes. Science Report. 2016;**6**:24922

[104] Li M, et al. An optimized procedure for exosome isolation and analysis using serum samples: Application to cancer biomarker discovery. Methods. 2015;**87**:26-30

[105] Drake RR, Kislinger T. The proteomics of prostate cancer exosomes. Expert Review of Proteomics. 2014;**11**(2):167-177

[106] Principe S, et al. In-depth proteomic analyses of exosomes isolated from expressed prostatic secretions in urine. Proteomics. 2013;**13**(10-11):1667-1671

[107] Dijkstra S, et al. Prostate cancer biomarker profiles in urinary sediments and exosomes. Journal of Urology. 2014;**191**(4):1132-1138

[108] Tanaka Y, et al. Clinical impact of serum exosomal microRNA-21 as a clinical biomarker in human esophageal squamous cell carcinoma. Cancer. 2013;**119**(6):1159-1167

[109] Wang H, et al. Expression of serum exosomal microRNA-21 in human hepatocellular carcinoma. Biomed Research International. 2014;**2014**:864894

[110] Liu J, et al. Increased exosomal microRNA-21 and microRNA-146a levels in the cervicovaginal lavage specimens of patients with cervical cancer. International Journal of Molecular Sciences. 2014;**15**(1):758-773

[111] Troyer DA, et al. A multicenter study shows PTEN deletion is strongly associated with seminal vesicle involvement and extracapsular extension in localized prostate cancer. Prostate. 2015;**75**(11):1206-1215

[112] Gabriel K, et al. Regulation of the tumor suppressor PTEN through exosomes: A diagnostic potential for prostate cancer. PLoS One. 2013;**8**(7):e70047

[113] Melo SA, et al. Glypican-1 identifies cancer exosomes and detects early pancreatic cancer. Nature. 2015;**523**(7559):177-182

[114] Consortium E-T, et al. EV-TRACK: Transparent reporting and centralizing knowledge in extracellular vesicle research. Nature Methods. 2017;**14**(3):228-232

Chapter 7

Microvesicles Released from Human Red Blood Cells: Properties and Potential Applications

Duc Bach Nguyen, Thi Bich Thuy Ly and
Ingolf Bernhardt

Additional information is available at the end of the chapter

http://dx.doi.org/10.5772/intechopen.69599

Abstract

Microvesicles (MVs) are small spherical fragments of plasma membrane between 50 and 1000 nm in diameter. MVs arise through direct outward budding and fission of the plasma membrane. As almost all cells, human red blood cells (RBCs) are able to release MVs into extracellular environment under stimulating or storage conditions. Recently, it has been known that MVs not only play a role in homeostasis but also have diverse functions in cell-cell interactions and in the pathogenesis of diseases. In this chapter, the formation and release of MVs from human RBCs have been described. In addition, MVs have demonstrated to be potential vehicle for transport of nucleic acid and other molecules to the target cells. Although RBC-derived MVs are potential material for the development of delivery systems, it is still a great challenge to the clinical application. Future research should pay more attention to MVs as biological targets for diagnosis and practical therapeutics of cancer and other diseases.

Keywords: microvesicles, red blood cell, exosomes, nucleic acid delivery, THP-1 cells, endothelial cells, transfection

1. Introduction

Extracellular vesicles (EVs) are spherical fragments released from biological membranes of various cell types under both physiological and pathological conditions. So far, many terms have been used to describe EVs, such as exosomes, microvesicles (MVs), membrane microparticles, ectosomes, and apoptotic bodies. Recently, based on their size and origin, EVs are classified as exosomes, MVs, and apoptotic bodies. Under stimulating or storage conditions, human red blood cells (RBCs) release EVs. This chapter focuses on the formation and release of MVs from human RBCs and considers the isolation and characterization of MVs in order to apply MVs as potential vehicles for nucleic acid delivery. Similar to EVs released from nucleated cells, MVs from human RBCs carry biomarkers originated from plasma membrane and also microRNAs but not DNA. These properties suggest that MVs can be used as potential vehicles to transport proteins, nucleic acids, or signal molecules. While the understanding of the biogenesis of MVs in human RBCs and their physiological role remains limited, accumulating data suggest that MVs may be applied in cancer therapy. This chapter reviews our current knowledge pertaining to MVs released from human RBCs. It describes the formation and biological properties of MVs and mentions the potential application of MVs as a molecular vehicle for drug and nucleic acid delivery. Furthermore, it gives an introduction in the application of MVs for cancer treatment. In addition, MVs and exosomes released from other cell types are also taken into consideration to provide findings of the nature of the membrane-derived vesicles, their mechanism of action, and their possible role in biological processes both under *in vitro* and *in vivo* conditions.

2. Microvesicles and their biological considerations

Under physiological and pathological conditions, various cell types release small spherical fragments called membrane vesicles or extracellular vehicles (EVs). So far, many different terms such as ectosomes, MVs, shedding vesicles, apoptosomes, membrane microparticles, or apoptotic bodies have been used in a vast number of reports on EVs [1–8]. Fifty years ago, in 1967, Wolf first identified small procoagulant structures deriving from activated platelets in human blood and created the initial term "platelet dust" [9]. Twenty years later, in 1987, Johnstone described the vesicle formation during maturation of sheep reticulocytes *in vitro* [10]. These findings were seen as a milestone in EV research allowing further studies on their function at various physiological conditions and in certain diseases. Since then, EVs have been detected in different body fluids such as peripheral blood, urine, saliva, semen, cerebrospinal fluid, synovial fluid, bronchoalveolar lavage, and bile. The mechanism of EV formation and the biochemical composition of EVs depend on cell types, physiological conditions, and the function of the cells from which they originate [11–16]. Recently, based on their size and biogenesis, EVs have been classified into exosomes, MVs, and apoptotic bodies. Exosomes are generally accepted to have size from 40 to 100 nm in diameter. They are secreted from endosomal compartments or multivesicular bodies of cells. In contrast, MVs including microparticles or membrane particles are larger in size varying from 50 to 1000 nm in diameter. The biogenesis of MVs arises through direct outward budding and fission of the plasma membrane following different kinds of cell activation or during early state of apoptosis [11, 17, 18]. Distinct from exosomes and MVs, apoptotic bodies are much larger with 1–5 μm in diameter. They are formed by cell-membrane blebbing when the cells undergo apoptosis [7, 11, 19–21]. Three subtypes of EVs, namely exosomes, MVs, and apoptotic bodies, are shown in **Figure 1**. In fact, it is still a challenge to separate one EV type from another because of their overlapping biophysical characteristics. Nevertheless, some discriminating markers have been reported [22]. In this chapter, the term MVs will be used for MVs, microparticles, or membrane microparticles (MPs) and EVs for both exosomes and MVs.

http://dx.doi.org/10.5772/intechopen.69599

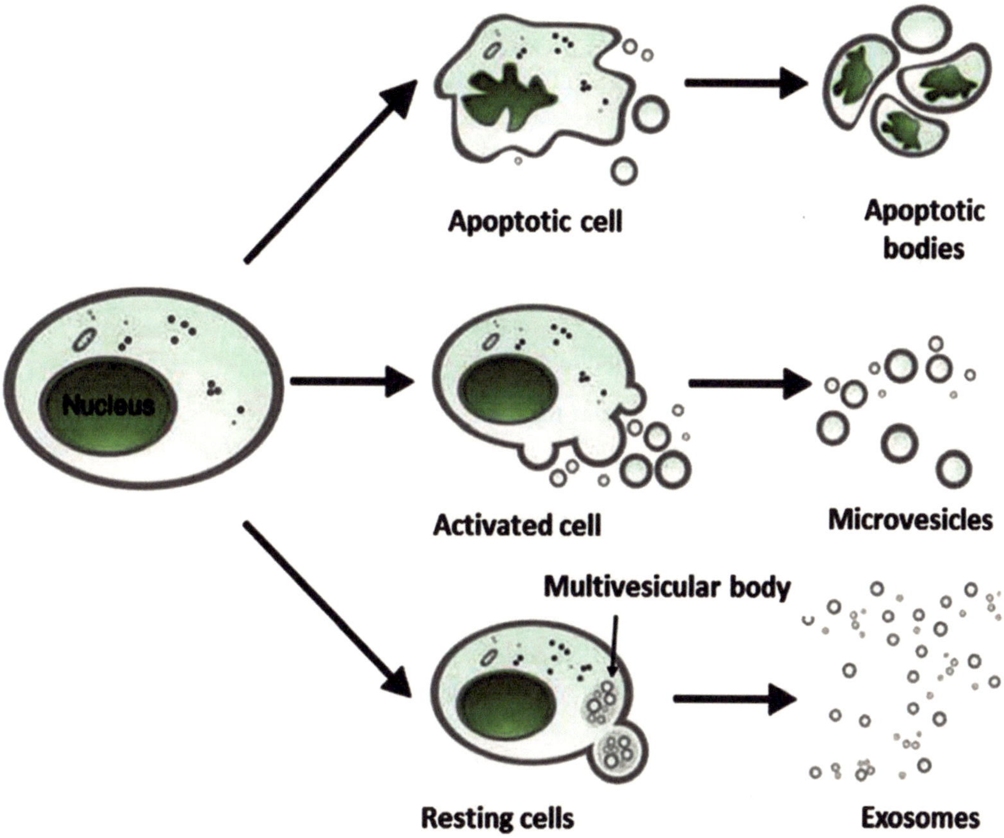

Figure 1. Potential vesicular structures of circulating DNA. Depending upon the mechanism of release, three subtypes of EVs, namely, exosomes, MVs, and apoptotic bodies, are described [28]. The figure is taken from Rykova et al. [29].

It has been reported that MVs are released from various types of activated or apoptotic cells including platelets, monocytes, endothelial cells (ECs), red blood cells, THP-1 monocytic cells, and granulocytes. MPs were also collected from the culture media, cell supernatants, and plasma by centrifugation at 20,000 g for 30 min. The average diameter of all types of MVs was varying much comparing different reports [19, 23–25]. The plasma MPs had the smallest size similar to MPs released from platelets and THP-1 cells, while MPs from monocytes were larger, and MPs from granulocytes and ECs were the largest ones. The data obtained from various reports indicate that the size of membrane MPs depends on the type of the cells from which they originate [23]. Although MVs have been discovered for years, the understanding of the mechanism of the formation as well as the biological roles of MVs is still a matter of debate. Recent reported findings led to advances of our understanding of the mechanism of formation and the role of MVs in many different diseases such as vascular diseases, cancer, infectious diseases, diabetes mellitus, diabetes, inflammation, and pathogen infection [24]. Inhibition of the production of MPs may serve as a novel therapeutic strategy for some diseases, especially for cancer treatment [11, 23, 26, 27]. In the next part of this chapter, the biogenesis, properties, and biological function of MVs released from human red blood cells (RBCs) are mainly addressed.

In the past decade, extracellular vesicles (EVs) have been recognized as potent vehicles of intercellular communication due to their capacity to transfer proteins, lipids, and nucleic acids, thereby influencing various physiological and pathological functions of both recipient and donor cells [30]. In addition, EVs also represent an important mode of intercellular communication by serving as vehicles for transfer between cells of membrane and cytosolic proteins, lipids, and RNA. Shortage of our knowledge of the molecular mechanisms for EV formation and lack of methods to interfere with the packaging of cargo or with vesicle release leads to a difficulty in identification of their physiological relevance *in vivo* [6]. EVs have been implicated in important biological processes such as surface-membrane trafficking and horizontal transfer of proteins and RNAs among neighboring cells, and distant tissues. Therefore, they play an important role in cell-to-cell communication under both physiological and disease conditions [11].

It is evident that direct investigation of the biological function of MVs *in vivo* is extremely complicated. Most of the studies regarding physiological roles of exosomes or MVs have to carry out *in vitro*, especially in the context of the immune system and cell-cell communication [31]. In 1996, a pioneering study by Raposo and colleagues demonstrated that exosomes derived from both human and mouse B-lymphocytes spread antigens bound to the class II major histocompatibility complex (MHC). These vesicle-associated complexes were capable of activating MHC class II leading to a restriction of T-cell responses. This finding suggests a role for exosomes in antigen presentation *in vivo* [32]. Furthermore, B cell–derived exosomes specifically interacted with the membrane of follicular dendritic cells derived from human tonsils. This finding is also an example for further supporting the idea of the active secretion of exosomes *in vivo* [33]. In addition, Montecalvo and colleagues demonstrated that different subsets of miRNAs are exchanged between follicular dendritic cells through exosomes at different maturation stages [34].

In a study, Wu showed that cancer cells release MVs and exosomes under both *in vivo* and *in vitro* conditions. MVs and exosomes carry different types of molecules on their surfaces, which are seen as biomarkers [24]. That is the reason why MVs or exosomes are used in cancer diagnosis. For example, circulating levels of MVs are elevated in gastric cancer patients. In these patients, MPs released from CD41a-positive platelets are significantly increased in stage IV compared with stage I or II/III [35]. It has been recently demonstrated that MVs released by cells represent another important mediator of cell-cell communication and are also an integral part of the intercellular microenvironment [3, 36, 37]. This opens a new scenario to understand signal and molecule transfers between cells even at long distances. For human RBCs, released MVs in both resting state (storage at 4°C) and stimulating conditions showed the ability to adhere together. It might be suggested that MVs are involved in the blot clot formation and also play a substantial role in the aggregation of stimulated RBCs [38, 39]. Further investigations have to be carried out to understand the role of MVs in both physiological and disease conditions.

It has been described that blood cells are able to generate a great variety of EVs. First identified in 1967, MVs are cell plasma membrane-derived small vesicles which are 0.1–1 mm in diameter. Later, the formation and release of EVs have been demonstrated in platelets, monocytes, endothelial cells, RBCs, and granulocytes [9]. EVs have been thought to serve as a disseminated storage pool of bio-effectors that circulate and play important roles in physiological homeostasis of the body under both physiological and disease conditions. Recent

http://dx.doi.org/10.5772/intechopen.69599

functional assays and analysis of MVs by multicolor flow cytometry have shown that MPs possess a broad spectrum of biological activities and may play an important role in multiple cellular processes including intercellular communication, immunity, apoptosis, and homeostasis [24, 40]. In case of human RBCs, MVs have a phospholipid bilayer structure exposing coagulant-active phosphatidylserine and expressing various membrane receptors [40]. It should be mentioned that mature human RBCs do not contain DNA but RNAs including mRNA and other non-coding RNAs. Therefore, it suggests that MVs from human RBCs may not only be involved in thrombosis, amplifying systemic inflammation or cell adhesion, but also in cell-cell interactions in term of nucleic acid transfer [38, 39, 41, 42].

Recently, it has been reported that negatively charged membranes of erythrocyte-derived microparticles display procoagulant activity [38, 39]. However, relatively little is known about the possible fibrinolytic activity of such MVs. This issue becomes particularly important during RBC storage, which significantly increases the number of MVs [43]. Regarding the ability of carrying nucleic acid, recently, a novel system composed of MVs from RBCs was created for efficient delivery of ultra-small superparamagnetic iron oxide particles into human bone marrow mesenchymal stem cells for cellular magnetic resonance imaging *in vitro* and *in vivo*. It showed that MVs are highly bio-safe to their autologous (exosomes) as manifested by cell viability, differentiation, and gene microarray assays. The data suggest that MVs could be used as potential intracellular delivery vehicles for biomedical applications [44]. More recently, a study of the function of MVs from human RBCs infected with *Plasmodium falciparum* parasites showed that infected RBC-derived MVs contain miRNAs that can modulate target genes in recipient cells. In addition, multiple miRNA species in EVs have been identified. They are bound to Ago2 and form functional complexes. The infected RBC-derived MVs were transfected successfully into endothelial cells repressing miRNA target genes and changed endothelial barrier properties [45]. In addition, role of RBCs-derived MVs in malaria response showed that the development of MVs by *Plasmodium sp*. has a major impact in disease outcomes and serves as an integral part in controlling stage switching in its life cycle. Clinical studies have highlighted elevated levels of EVs in patients with severe malaria disease, and EVs have been linked to increased sequestration of infected RBCs to the endothelium [46].

3. Formation and release of MVs from human red blood cells

It has been known that during their 120-day of lifespan, RBCs lose approximately 20% of their volume through vesicle release, whereas their hemoglobin concentration increases by 14% [47]. Although a number of mechanisms explaining the formation of MVs have been proposed, the creation and the role of RBC microparticles are far from being completely understood. It has been pronounced that the formation of MVs involves the activity of certain components of the plasma membrane as well as cytoskeletal proteins [19]. Under physiological conditions, the phospholipids of the cell membrane are distributed asymmetrically. In particular, phosphatidylcholine (PC) and sphingomyelin (SM) are predominantly present in the outer membrane leaflet, while phosphatidylserine (PS) and phosphatidylethanolamine (PE) are located predominantly in the inner membrane leaflet. This asymmetric distribution is controlled by a group of enzymes, flippase, floppase, and scramblase [48–51]. The flippase is responsible for the transfer of PE and PS from the outer to the inner leaflet of the cell membrane, while the floppase has been shown to have the opposite effect. Their activity is regulated by ABCC1 protein, also known as a multidrug-resistant protein 1 [19]. In contrast, the distribution of the phospholipid PS is determined by the activity of the scramblase. In human RBCs, the mechanism of the formation of MVs has been investigated and described by many research groups [50–54].

The integrity of RBC membrane is supported from many components of cytoskeleton structure, e.g., hexagonal actin–spectrin lattice anchoring with other proteins such as glycophorin A and band 3 protein [55]. It has been described that the vesiculation would be a mean for RBCs to get rid of specific harmful agents such as denatured hemoglobin, C5b-9 complement attack complex, band 3 neoantigen, and IgG that tend to accumulate in RBCS or on their membrane during their lifespan [22]. An influx of Ca^{2+} through nonspecific cation channels leads to the activation of several enzymes such as calpain or scramblase leading to the externalization of phosphatidylserine of the RBC membrane and degradation of cytoskeleton proteins and aggregation of band 3 leading to vesiculation [41, 56]. In our recent study, the kinetics of membrane blebbing and formation of MVs were characterized by using annexin V-FITC and fluorescence microscopy. The kinetics of budding and shedding of MVs were captured in every 30 s. Treatment of RBCs with a calcium inonophore (as positive control), lysophosphatidic acid (LPA), or phorbol-12-myristate-13-acetate (PMA) led to the externalization of PS at the outer membrane leaflet of RBCs as well released MVs. Moreover, it was interesting to see that a stimulation of RBCs by PMA in the absence of Ca^{2+} also led to the release of MVs [17, 41]. This suggests that the formation of MVs is also under the control of a calcium-independent pathway related to the activity of the PKC (**Figure 2**).

Based on the current understanding, a scheme with the interaction of protein components in the cells has been proposed. The proposed mechanism for the budding and shedding of MVs in human RBCs is shown in **Figure 3**.

Although many factors influence the formation and release of MVs, Ca^{2+} and PKC play essential roles in the process of MV formation [17, 19, 41]. An increase of intracellular calcium inactivates the flippase and activates the scramblase as well as the floppase leading to a reorganization of phospholipids in the cell membrane [21, 22, 41, 53, 54, 57]. The activation of calpain and degradation of actin filaments leads to breaking of bonds between the cytoskeleton filaments and the phospholipids. The weakening of the protein fibrils of the cytoskeleton initiates the budding and shedding of MVs [52, 58–60]. It has been demonstrated that reorganization or disruption of the cytoskeleton plays an important role in the release of MVs [36]. Another study showed that the activation of the scramblase requires a larger increase of the calcium concentration and therefore it is considered as being less important for the formation of MVs [19, 50]. By using a special compound R5421, a scramblase-specific inhibitor, it has been shown that vesicle shedding was attenuated in human RBCs [52, 61]. By adding ascorbic acid to RBCs during storage, a significant decrease in MVs formation was observed [62]. In our study, the MVs formation was observed within 1 hour when RBCs were treated with the PKC activator, phorbol-12-myristate-13-acetate (PMA), even in the absence of Ca^{2+}. In addition, the kinetics of the formation of MVs in human RBCs has recently investigated by real-time measurement using fluorescence microscopy [17].

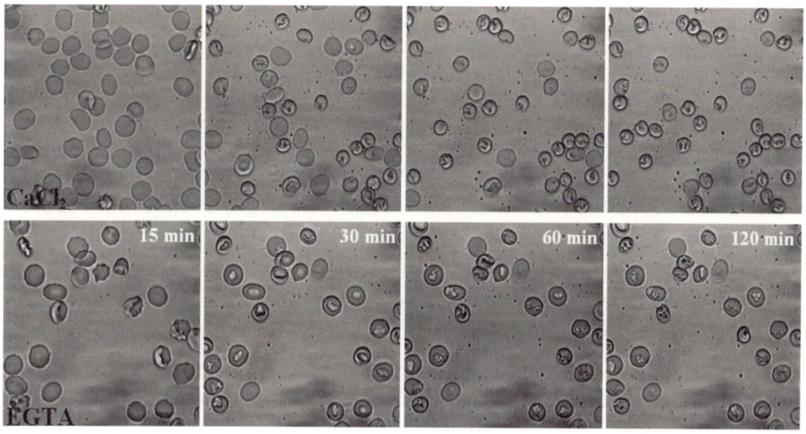

Figure 2. Bright field imaging of the formation of MVs in human RBCs depending on time (up to 120 min) stimulated by 6 μM PMA in the presence of 2 mM Ca^{2+} (upper row) and in the absence of Ca^{2+} and with 2 mM EGTA (lower row).

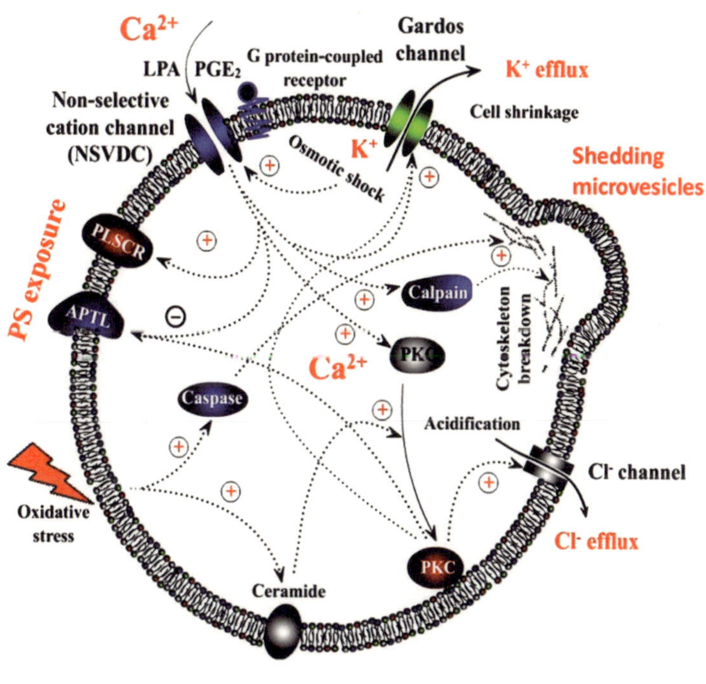

Figure 3. Proposed mechanisms of the formation of MVs in human RBCs. Lysophosphatidic acid (LPA) or prostaglandin E2 (PGE2), which are two typical substances released from activated platelets, activate a nonselective voltage-dependent cation (NSVDC) channel. The opening of this channel leads to an increase of the intracellular Ca^{2+} content. An increase of the intracellular Ca^{2+} level activates the phospholipid scramblase (PLSCR) and the protein kinase C (PKC). The activated PKC moves from the cytoplasma to the membrane. The amino-phospholipid translocase (APLT) is inhibited by high concentrations of intracellular Ca^{2+}, PKC, and ATP depletion. The PKC also activates and opens Cl^- channels leading to an efflux of Cl^-. The efflux of Cl^- leads to an intracellular acidification. Under stress conditions, ceramide is formed and caspases are activated. Calpains are a family of calcium-dependent non-lysosomal cysteine proteases activated by Ca^{2+}. When caspase and calpain are activated, they are able to break down the cytoskeleton by a proteolysis activity leading to membrane blebbing and vesicle formation [41].

4. Content and biomarkers of microvesicles

4.1. Content of microvesicles

In recent years, numerous works have focused on providing a comprehensive characterization of the content of exosomes and MVs. Recently, information about molecules including proteins, mRNAs, microRNAs, or lipids observed within these vesicles has been deposited in EVpedia and Vesiclepedia [48, 63, 64]. By the end of 2015, Vesiclepedia stores records for 92,897 proteins, 27,642 mRNAs, 4934 miRNAs, and 584 lipids from 538 studies in 33 different species [48]. These numbers suggest that exosomes and MVs contain an extremely broad and heterogeneous range of molecules. Although these databases are extremely valuable, it still needs more evidences to elucidate the biological role of MVs and exosomes because the processes of biogenesis and packing molecules into these vesicles are complicated. It should be also mentioned here that the interpretation of the content of exosomes and MVs may be influenced or interfered by artifacts in sample preparation, isolation procedures, and analysis methods [65]. In comparison to MVs, exosomes are vesicles secreted upon fusion of multivesicular endosomes with the cell surface. Thus, exosomes transfer not only membrane components but also nucleic acid among different cells. Therefore, in order to understand the function of exosomes, it is necessary to have more evidences at subcellular compartments and mechanisms involved in the biogenesis and secretion of these vesicles [66]. Moreover, for many years, it is commonly thought that human mature RBCs do not contain nucleic acids because they are terminally differentiated cells without nuclei and organelles. However, transcriptomic analysis of a purified population of human mature RBCs from individuals with normal hemoglobin (HbAA) and homozygous sickle cell disease (HbSS) showed that there was a significant difference in microRNA expression in HbAA in comparison with HbSS [67]. This finding is very important to understand that MVs released from human mature RBCs carry nucleic acid and are likely involved in the biological processes of cell-cell communication and nucleic acid delivery.

4.2. Biomarkers on microvesicles

It is known that the antigens occurring on MVs are typical for cells from which the MVs are released. Depending on the origin of formation, MVs contain numerous markers that determine their origin, e.g., CD41 for platelets, CD235a and Ter-119 for RBCs [55, 68], and CD11c for dendritic cells [69]. Additionally, MVs released from B cells, dendritic cells, and melanoma cell lines are richer in sphingomyelin, rather than in cholesterol which are also characteristics of their parental cells [70]. Some glycoproteins on the surface of RBCs expressed at low and variable levels protect RBCs from damage and elimination. These include complement inhibitors, such as DAF and CD59, and signaling molecules such as CD47 [71, 72] and SHPS-1, a multifunctional transmembrane glycoprotein [72]. These makers inhibit phagocytosis of RBCs by macrophages because CD47 prevents this elimination by binding to the inhibitory receptor signal regulatory protein alpha (SIRPα) [73]. Therefore, these markers also exist on the surfaces of MVs released from RBCs [11, 74, 75]. In human RBCs, if the released MVs carry CD47 on their surface, they may be avoided from the clearance by macrophages [76, 77].

Studies on proteomics of MVs released from human RBCs were first carried out by Bosman presenting pioneering investigations [78–80]. In these series of studies, membranes of intact RBCs and MVs were compared, allowing the identification of several proteins differentially expressed between the two types of samples. Together with further studies on the oxidation and the depletion of spectrins and cytoskeletal proteins such as proteins 4.1 and 4.2, band 3 followed by the time course of storage, it has been concluded that RBCs have the ability to get rid of harmful materials by vesiculation such as denatured hemoglobin, C5b-9 complement attack complex, and band 3 neoantigen [81, 82]. In human RBCs, the formation of MVs has been described as part of the RBC senescence process [47, 78] and also proposed as part of an apoptosis-like form of these cells [20, 21].

It should be also mentioned that due to the variation of the lateral composition of the cell membrane, MVs originated from the same cell may contain different proteins or lipid components. Proteomic analyses have revealed that the spectrum of proteins found in MVs released from cultured cells is influenced partly by the stimulating conditions, which were used to trigger the vesiculation [36]. A study on the components of proteins in human RBC-derived MVs by two-dimensional gel electrophoresis discovered that the protein components in MVs under various stimulating conditions (cold storage and increased intracellular calcium level) are different. This was especially the case for sorcin, grancalcin, PDCD6, and particularly annexins IV and V [83]. Therefore, the molecular pathways to form MVs are different under both *in vivo* and *in vitro* conditions. In addition, this finding suggests that MVs may be also classified based on the presence of proteins. Recently, a method has been reported using carboxyfluorescein diacetate succinimidyl ester, which allows to detect the phospholipid component PS in the outer membrane leaflet of MVs that fail to react with annexin V [84]. This study is very important for screening blood products during storage in blood bank because the formation of MVs with PS in the outer membrane leaflet may lead to thrombus formation or aggregation of RBCs or phagocytosis.

It seems relatively simple to isolate EVs from human plasma with available protocols described elsewhere. However, to isolate MVs from RBCs, it requires a step to separate only RBCs without contamination of platelets or white cells. Upon the purpose of study, MVs can be collected by differential centrifugation. Menck and colleagues isolated and distinguished MVs and exosome from human blood cells using Western blot analysis. The data revealed that MVs pelleted from EDTA-anticoagulated plasma samples by differential centrifugation were 100–600 nm in diameter. MVs can be distinguished from exosomes by detecting the presence of proteins tubulin, actinin-4, or mitofilin, while antibodies for CD9 and CD81 were used as markers for exosomes [85].

5. Stability of microvesicles

Jayachandran and colleagues isolated MVs from platelet-free plasma (PFP) and platelet poor plasmas (PPP) and stored the MVs at either −40 or −80°C for more than a year. No effect on MV counts irrespective of initial counts was observed after three freeze thaw cycles of PFP [86]. Another investigation on the stability of MVs after different times of storage at 4 and

−80°C by using flow cytometry analysis showed that there was no significant difference by counts and size distribution of MVs stored at 4°C for 3–4 days or 1 week and MVs frozen at −80°C for 1 or 4 weeks [87]. In another study, Gallart showed that plasma containing exosomes and MVs frozen at −150°C can keep vesicles intact for long time [88]. Investigation was carried on the effect of short-term storage and temperature on the stability of exosome by incubating at temperatures ranging from −70 to 90°C for 30 min. Immunoblot results showed that all exosome-associated proteins incubated at 90°C were mostly degraded for a short period of time. The effect of long-term storage was carried out by incubating isolated exosomes for 10 days at wide range of temperature from −70°C to room temperature (RT). It revealed that protein and RNA amounts were significantly reduced at RT compared with data obtained at −70 and 4°C. Incubation at 4°C and RT resulted in major loss of CD63, and decreasing level of HSP70 was shown only at RT. In addition, flow cytometry result showed that exosome population became more dispersed after RT incubation for 10 days compared with −70°C incubated or freshly isolated exosomes [88]. Study on exosomes isolated from urine defined that freezing at −20°C caused a major loss of the integrity of these exosomes. In contrast, storage at −80°C increased the recovery almost complete (86%). Vortexing after thawing resulted in a significantly increased recovery of exosomes in urine frozen at −20 or −80°C, even if it was frozen for 7 months [89]. A similar study has been done to evaluate the stability of MVs released in whole blood samples under the influence of different anticoagulants. Analysis of MVs stored at 4°C and RT using nanoparticle tracking analysis (NTA) showed that total MV counts increased after 24 hours in sodium citrated or heparinized blood. The presence of EDTA showed stable platelet-derived MVs and RBC-derived MV counts at RT over a period of 48 h [90].

6. Isolation and characterization of microvesicles

Currently, there is no standard protocol for isolation of EVs for either therapeutic application or basic research [91]. However, a conventional method to obtain EVs is ultrafiltration followed by differential centrifugation. Ultrafiltration and size-exclusion liquid chromatography is suitable for EV isolation at large scale [92]. In fact, many research groups use differential centrifugation combined with filtration to isolate and define the MVs or exosomes. For example, a centrifugation force from 10,000 to 20,000 g is commonly applied to pellet MVs and from 70,000 to 100,000 g or even higher for exosomes. Although the centrifuge force is indicated in a number of publications, it is still varying among research groups. Nevertheless, there is always an overlap in the size of collected MVs or exosomes when analyzed by using dynamic light scattering (DLS) method. Therefore, the procedure for sample preparation and also isolation of MVs should be simplified as much as possible with minimal steps. In general, four critical steps should be taken into consideration: (i) removal of intact cells and large cell debris by low-speed centrifugation of the extracellular fluid (200–1000 g for 3–15 min); (ii) pelleting of large, secreted vesicles from the cell-free supernatant by medium-speed centrifugation (10,000 g for 30 min, a minimum of 2 times); (iii) collection of small, secreted vesicles by ultracentrifugation at 70,000–100,000 g, and (iv) noting all other parameters and type of rotors used in experiments [7].

At present, there is still a lack of studies assessing EV products after periods of storage. However, our unpublished investigations showed that the polydispersity (PI) of MV increased proportionally with the storage time at −20°C in deionized water. Vortexing was useful to recover MVs after storage. Further studies have to be done investigating the stability and the polydispersity of MVs in different solvents or buffers. The results of such analyses will facilitate defining provisional shelf-life times of EV-based products. The materials used for sample preparation, isolation, and storage should also be taken into consideration, especially for human therapeutics because solvents and buffers have a strong influence on the stability of EVs, especially after storage [93]. There is a wide range of solvents from water, sodium chloride solution, to phosphate-buffered saline (PBS), Tris-HCl, HEPES, and glycerol. However, glycerol and dimethyl sulfoxide (DMSO) showed a significant influence to the stability of EVs [94]. For investigation of the function and physical properties of EVs, isotonic buffers are recommended to prevent pH shifts during storage as well as during freezing and thawing procedures. Although PBS or other phosphate-containing buffers are widely used, it has to be considered to avoid calcium even at a very low concentration due to the formation of calcium phosphate aggregated in the buffer as nanoparticles, which can interfere with EV quantification assays [93]. Storage vials can also affect the quality of EVs due to unexpected or irreversible binding to certain materials. Thus, vials should be carefully selected to eliminate the factors that influence the concentration or integrity of stored EVs [93, 95].

So far, a variety of techniques have been commonly used to study MVs released from human RBCs. Traditionally, nanoparticle analysis is available to analyze the particles at nanosize including flow cytometry, DLS, and electron microscopy. Most widespread is flow cytometry; however, commercial flow cytometry typically has a lower practical size limit (for polystyrene beads) of around 300 nm at which point the signal is hard to distinguish clearly from the baseline noise level or so-called "dust" [96]. Fluorescence labeling can be efficient to detect particles at lower sizes. DLS has also been used, but being an ensemble measurement, the results comprise either a simple z-average (intensity weighted) particle size and polydispersity (PI), or a very limited-resolution particle size distribution profile. Electron microscopy is a useful research tool for studying micro- and nanovesicles but at high running costs and extensive sample preparation [22]. Atomic force microscope (AFM) is also an applicable method to measure the size and also the morphology of MVs [17]. An alternative approach for measuring EVs is using the NTA method. In NTA, the size is derived from the measurement of Brownian motion of EVs in a liquid suspension [22].

In recent study, under stimulating conditions, MVs from RBCs were collected by differential centrifugation and characterized by using SEM, AFM, and DLS. Data from the measurement using a Zetasizer (Nano ZS) for both size and zeta potential showed that the sizes of two subpopulations of MVs were 125.6 ± 31.4 nm and 205.8 ± 51.4 nm. There was an overlapping in the size of the two populations in the region from 150 to 200 nm. Zeta potential of released MVs was measured in different solvents showing negative values from −40 to −10 mV depending on the solvent used [17]. The morphology and size of MVs released from human RBCs were also analyzed using AFM and SEM (**Figure 4**).

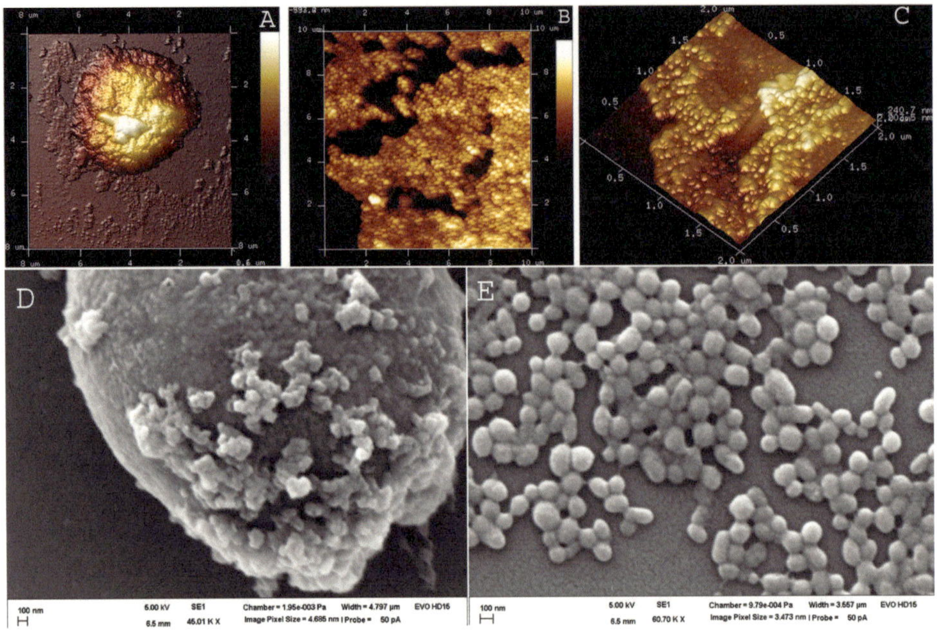

Figure 4. Topographical imaging of stimulated RBCs and released MVs. Glutaraldehyde-fixed samples of PMA-stimulated RBCs using AFM (A) and SEM (D); MVs scanning using AFM (B, C) and SEM (E) [17].

7. Potential applications of microvesicles

The structural feature that makes EVs especially attractive for drug delivery purpose is due to their analogy to liposomes. This means that EVs originated from an organism can be used as conventional liposome with an advantage when they are administered to the same organism *in vivo*. EVs are able to deliver molecules through hard-to-cross barriers like the blood-brain barrier. Therefore, EVs can be used for loading with drugs or other bioactive molecules and then work as efficient delivery systems. Several strategies are described for loading small molecule and genetic materials into liposomes; however, most of these strategies are not feasible for exosomes [97–99]. Two major strategies have been applied to load small molecules or drugs to EVs. The first possibility is the loading after EV isolation, and the second is the loading during EV biogenesis. In addition to loading, labeling of MVs is required to detect or investigate the efficiency of delivery to target cells and the expression of protein or function of miRNAs in recipient cells. So far, several techniques and methods have been applied to label MVs. Most common methods are incubation with fluorescence lipophilic dye, biotinylated radioisotope, substrate of luciferase (for *in vivo* trial), streptavidin-conjugated fluorescence dyes, or other modified proteins [100].

7.1. Microvesicles and nucleic acid transport

When nucleic acid (DNA, RNA) is directly introduced to the body, it will be rapidly removed out of the circulation via degradation by nucleases or by kidneys before reaching the target tissues or cells of interest. Recent evidence has shown that different kinds of RNAs are transported by EVs during cell-cell communications. It has been shown that miRNAs are enriched in EVs in form of miRNA-RISC complexes and transferred from exosomes and MVs to many different cells. As such, EVs can be applied as a new attractive alternative approach for therapeutic miRNA delivery [14]. Recently, a study showed that embryonic stem cell MVs likely are useful therapeutic tools for transferring mRNA, microRNAs, protein, and siRNA to cells and also important mediators of signaling within stem cell niches [101]. It has been known that the lipids, proteins, mRNA, and microRNA (miRNA) delivered by these vesicles change the phenotype of the receiving cells [11, 102]. The ability to encapsulate and deliver different types of nucleic acid of both exosomes and MVs has been investigated. The results showed that MVs delivered functional plasmid DNA, but not RNA, whereas exosomes from the same source did not deliver functional nucleic acids. These results have significant implications for understanding the role of EVs in cellular communication and also the role of MVs for development of tools for nucleic acid delivery [11]. MVs from human RBCs infected with *P. falciparum* parasites contain miRNAs that can modulate target genes in recipient endothelial cells and serve as an integral part in controlling stage switching in the life cycle of the parasites [45, 46]. A typical example of application of EVs as vehicle for drug transport is the loading of curcumin, chemotherapeutic compounds paclitaxel and doxorubicin to EVs using electroporation. After transfecting loaded EVs to implanted breast tumor tissues, the results showed that the loaded EVs suppressed the growth of tumors without causing any toxicity [103]. As such, curcumin-loaded EVs have already made their way into the clinic to specifically suppress the activation of myeloid cells [93, 104].

7.2. Transfection of nucleic acid mediated by microvesicles

The strategy for cancer treatments is specifically killing malignant cells by vehicles, which carry appropriate substances or compounds to the target cells. Unfortunately, so far, it was not successful to cure the disease. The current concept in tumor treatment is to control the microenvironment of the tumor because the tumor is not only composed of malignant cells but also consists of other groups of cells that work together [105, 106]. Future research directions should draw more attention to EVs as biological targets for diagnosis, prognosis, and therapy of cancer. In addition, EVs participate and play a significant role in cell communication, and therefore they may become a valuable drug delivery system [107]. So far, a vast number of investigation on exosomes in carrying and transport of nucleic acid to target cells have been carried out; however, more information about using MVs to carry nucleic acid for transfection to cultured cells is required. Recently, an investigation of the capacity of MVs to deliver functional nucleic acids was carried out by using recipient HEK293FT cells cultured with exosomes and MVs derived from transfected donor cells with the fusion protein Luc–RFP as reporter. The data revealed that only loaded MVs led to Luc–RFP expression in the recipient HEK293FT cells, even though both MVs and exosomes encapsulated the reporter proteins. After the MV-mediated transfer, the bioluminescence signal increased over 3 days that was not observed in case of exosomes. The finding suggested that nucleic acids were delivered and led to a *de novo* expression of reporter proteins in recipient HEK293FT cells. By comparison with HEK293FT cells transfected by lipofectin with Luc-encoding pDNA, there was a different time course of Luc expression of the two methods. This observation suggested that the mechanism of MV-mediated delivery of nucleic acids and protein expression may be different from that of cationic liposome-based delivery of pDNA, which is typically used for transfection to culture cells [11]. Although this finding was very important to confirm the ability of MVs in carrying nucleic acid and transfection to recipient KEK293FT cells, experiments with different cell types are required. Another example is the study using MVs shed from the monocytic cell line THP-1 enriched with miR-150 to transfect to endothelial cells promoting angiogenesis of these cells [108]. MicroRNA-223 delivered by platelet-derived MVs promotes lung cancer cell invasion via targeting tumor suppressor EPB41L3 [109]. Another example of using MVs in nucleic acid delivery was the work of Zhang to prove the inhibitory effect of TGF-β1 siRNA delivered by mouse fibroblast L929 cell-derived MVs (L929 MVs) on the growth and metastasis of murine sarcomas 180 cells both *in vitro* and *in vivo*. By comparing to the same concentration of free TGF-β1 siRNA, TGF-β1 siRNA delivered by L929 MVs efficiently decreased the level of TGF-β1 in the recipient tumor cells [110]. Other works dealing with miR-150 proved that MVs can be an excellent carrier for nucleic acid delivery [108, 110]. Taken all together, MVs carrying microRNAs can influence the recipient cell phenotypes.

7.3. Efficiency of nucleic acid transfection by microvesicles

Protein expression induced by MV-mediated pDNA delivery is a slower process than after transfection using cationic lipid complexes. It may be due to that fact that loaded MV need to fuse with the endosomal membrane before releasing nucleic acid contents into the cytosol. Studies on EVs from transiently transfected cells may be confounded by a predominance of pDNA transfer. Compare the efficiency of transfection of MVs loaded with pDNA or RNA, it revealed that MVs functionally deliver DNA much better than RNA. Further studies of the nature of this transfer are necessary to understand the specificity of pDNA loading pathways and delivery mechanisms [11]. So far, small RNAs have been successfully loaded into MVs for a variety of delivery applications; however, the potential use of MVs for DNA delivery has been abandoned. By using electroporation, Lamichhane investigated the ability of loading MVs with linear DNA. Loading efficiency and capacity of DNA in MVs were dependent on DNA size as well as on the conformation of DNA. By using this approach, linear DNA molecules with less than 1000 bp in length were more efficiently associated with MVs compared to larger linear DNAs and pDNA. In addition, MV size was also influencing the potential of DNA loading, as larger MVs encapsulated more linear and plasmid DNA than smaller vesicles and exosomes. These results demonstrated critical parameters that define the potential use of MVs for gene therapy [111]. Another example is the application of EVs isolated from media of cultured cardiomyocytes derived from adult mouse heart. These EVs, which were transfected to target fibroblasts, led to a change in the gene expression patterns in comparison with controls [112]. Recently, a study on delivery of a therapeutic mRNA or protein via MVs for treatment of cancer was carried out. Genetically engineered MVs by expressing high levels of the suicide gene mRNA and protein–cytosine deaminase (CD) fused to uracil phosphoribosyl transferase (UPRT) in MV from HEK-293T cells. Isolated MVs from these cells were used to treat pre-established nerve sheath tumors (schwannomas) in a mouse model. MV-mediated delivery of CD-UPRT mRNA or protein by direct injection into schwannomas led to regression of these tumors. This finding suggests that MVs can serve as novel cell-derived vehicle to effectively deliver therapeutic mRNA/proteins for treatment of diseases [113]. Taken all together, the results from these studies suggest that MVs can be used as new vehicles for nucleic acid transfer.

7.4. Development of microvesicle-based delivery systems

Although EVs were applied to humans already in the early 2000s for the treatment of cancer patients, no recommended standard techniques have been established for the production of EVs at clinical grade. Several manufacturing and safety considerations need to be addressed and appropriate quality controls have to be implemented and validated. It remains a challenge to set up platforms for the production of EVs at clinical grade that fulfill all necessary criteria for the successful approval of subsequent EV-based clinical trials [93]. The most relevant issue to be addressed at the various levels of the developmental processes is to bring MV-based therapeutics into the clinical application in treatment of diseases including cancers. It is obvious that MVs are part of parental plasma cells; therefore, their antigenicity is mainly determined by protein and lipid components, profile of miRNAs and mRNAs, and also other factors originated from the parent's cells. Similar to exosomes, MVs are able to overcome limitations of cell-based therapeutics including safety, manufacturing, and availability. With a capability of crossing the blood-brain barrier, which classically acts as a major hurdle in the administration of therapeutic agents for targeting cells and tissue, especially of the central nervous system, MVs can be applied for the transport of molecules to target cells or tissues [114, 115] The presence of biomarkers on the surface may drive the loaded MVs to the specific target and help them to protect their cargoes from degradation [65, 116]. The standard procedure for isolation, purification, and storage of EVs at large scale should be established for certain cell types for trials at both *in vitro* and *in vivo* levels.

Another important issue in application of MVs is how to load bioactive compounds into these vesicles. For example, in order to load MVs with therapeutic small RNA molecules, two encapsulation approaches commonly used are post-loading or pre-loading. Post-loading method is using a specific method to introduce RNA into EVs (e.g., electroporation) while pre-loading is carried out during the EV formation (it is also called endogenous method that exploits the cellular machinery for small RNA loading into EVs). This endogenous method has been successfully used for the packaging of both siRNA and miRNA in EVs [99, 117, 118]. Functional delivery into recipient cells has been shown in several reports [119–121]. Several recent reports have shown functional siRNA delivery into recipient cells using EVs loaded by electroporation. However, the efficacy of this exogenous method has not been fully demonstrated, and other research groups stated that the loading of EVs with miRNA by using this method was not successful [120, 122]. Therefore, further studies are needed to confirm the feasibility and efficiency of this method for EVs loading. Nevertheless, the feasibility of the method likely varies depending on the siRNA or miRNA species. Furthermore, the efficiency of the overexpression or the direct transfection of particular small RNA-loaded EVs to recipient cells is still the matter of concern.

8. Conclusion

MVs are able to carry macromolecules, especially nucleic acid, and play a key role in cellular communication. In near future, MVs may efficiently support for the conventional treatment of tumor or cancer, which are using chemotherapeutic drugs, radiation therapy, or surgery.

Recent findings suggest that released MVs from human RBCs can be applied as novel treatment for various diseases including cancer. Structurally, MVs contain various membrane receptors and also carry nucleic acids, proteins, or other molecules. With many advantages in overcoming many of the limitations of cell-based therapeutics including safety, manufacturing, and availability, MVs may serve as cell-to-cell shuttles for carrying bioactive molecules to target cells. Therefore, MVs involve biological processes, especially the interaction with tumors or cancers. Human RBCs, with a large number of cells in the human body, can be easily collected without requiring cell culturing or sophisticated instrumentation. In addition, MVs released from RBCs can move to almost all tissues in the body without being hindered by any biological barrier. Therefore, MVs from human RBCs are potential candidates for the transport of nucleic acid and other bioactive compounds to the target cells. However, to make MVs to become applicable and efficacious in therapeutic treatments, underlying functions of MVs still need to be better understood. Future research directions should pay more attention to MVs as biological targets for cancer diagnosis, prognosis, and therapy that enable MVs as new source and of new material and promising approach for practical therapeutics.

Acknowledgements

The authors would like to thank the Vietnam National Foundation for Science and Technology Development (NAFOSTED) for the support under the grant number 106-YS.06-2013.16. Nguyen Duc Bach received this grant including the travel expenses for working in the group of IB.

Author details

Duc Bach Nguyen[1*], Thi Bich Thuy Ly[2] and Ingolf Bernhardt[3]

*Address all correspondence to: ndbach@vnua.edu.vn

1 Department of Molecular Biology, Faculty of Biotechnology, Vietnam National University of Agriculture, Hanoi, Vietnam

2 Institute of Biotechnology, Vietnam Academy of Science and Technology, Hanoi, Vietnam

3 Laboratory of Biophysics, Saarland University, Saarbruecken, Germany

References

[1] Holme PA, Solum NO, Brosstad F, Roger M, Abdelnoor M. Demonstration of platelet-derived microvesicles in blood from patients with activated coagulation and fibrinolysis using a filtration technique and western blotting. Thrombosis and Haemostasis. 1994;**72**(5):666-671

[2] Hess C, Sadallah S, Hefti A, Landmann R, Schifferli JA. Ectosomes released by human neutrophils are specialized functional units. Journal of Immunology. 1999;**163**(8):4564-4573

[3] Cocucci E, Racchetti G, Meldolesi J. Shedding microvesicles: Artefacts no more. Trends in Cell Biology. 2009;**19**(2):43-51

[4] Gyorgy B, Szabo TG, Pasztoi M, Pal Z, Misjak P, Aradi B, et al. Membrane vesicles, current state-of-the-art: Emerging role of extracellular vesicles. Cellular and Molecular Life Sciences. 2011;**68**(16):2667-2688

[5] Trams EG, Lauter CJ, Salem Jr N, Heine U. Exfoliation of membrane ecto-enzymes in the form of micro-vesicles. Biochimica et Biophysica Acta. 1981;**645**(1):63-70

[6] Raposo G, Stoorvogel W. Extracellular vesicles: Exosomes, microvesicles, and friends. Journal of Cell Biology. 2013;**200**(4):373-383

[7] Gould SJ, Raposo G. As we wait: Coping with an imperfect nomenclature for extracellular vesicles. Journal of Extracellular Vesicles. 2013;**2**(2)

[8] Zaborowski MP, Balaj L, Breakefield XO, Lai CP. Extracellular vesicles: Composition, biological relevance, and methods of study. Bioscience. 2015;**65**(8):783-797

[9] Wolf P. The nature and significance of platelet products in human plasma. British Journal of Haematology. 1967;**13**(3):269-288

[10] Johnstone RM, Adam M, Hammond JR, Orr L, Turbide C. Vesicle formation during reticulocyte maturation. Association of plasma membrane activities with released vesicles (exosomes). Journal of Biological Chemistry. 1987;**262**(19):9412-9420

[11] Kanada M, Bachmann MH, Hardy JW, Frimannson DO, Bronsart L, Wang A, et al. Differential fates of biomolecules delivered to target cells via extracellular vesicles. Proceedings of the National Academy of Sciences of the United States of America. 2015;**112** (12):E1433-1442

[12] Freyssinet JM, Toti F. Formation of procoagulant microparticles and properties. Thrombosis Research. 2010;**125** Suppl 1(1):S46-48

[13] Frydrychowicz M, Kolecka-Bednarczyk A, Madejczyk M, Yasar S, Dworacki G. Exosomes - structure, biogenesis and biological role in non-small-cell lung cancer. Scandinavian Journal of Immunology. 2015;**81**(1):2-10

[14] Lee Y, El Andaloussi S, Wood MJ. Exosomes and microvesicles: Extracellular vesicles for genetic information transfer and gene therapy. Human Molecular Genetics. 2012;**21** (R1):R125-134

[15] Horstman LL, Ahn YS. Platelet microparticles: A wide-angle perspective. Critical Reviews in Oncology Hematology. 1999;**30**(2):111-142

[16] Flaumenhaft R. Formation and fate of platelet microparticles. Blood Cells Molecules and Diseases. 2006;**36**(2):182-187

[17] Nguyen DB, Ly TB, Wesseling MC, Hittinger M, Torge A, Devitt A, et al. Characterization of microvesicles released from human red blood cells. Cellular Physiology and Biochemistry. 2016;**38**(3):1085-1099

[18] Inal JM, Kosgodage U, Azam S, Stratton D, Antwi-Baffour S, Lange S. Blood/plasma secretome and microvesicles. Biochimica et Biophysica Acta. 2013;**1834**(11):2317-2325

[19] Zmigrodzka M, Guzera M, Miskiewicz A, Jagielski D, Winnicka A. The biology of extracellular vesicles with focus on platelet microparticles and their role in cancer development and progression. Tumor Biology. 2016;**37**(11):14391-14401

[20] Foller M, Huber SM, Lang F. Erythrocyte programmed cell death. International Union of Biochemistry and Molecular Biology Life. 2008;**60**(10):661-668

[21] Lang F, Gulbins E, Lerche H, Huber SM, Kempe DS, Foller M. Eryptosis, a window to systemic disease. Cellular Physiology and Biochemistry. 2008;**22**(5-6):373-380

[22] Tissot J-D, Canellini G, Rubin O, Angelillo-Scherrer A, Delobel J, Prudent M, Lion N. Blood microvesicles: From proteomics to physiology. Translational Proteomics. 2013;**1**(1): 38-52

[23] Alchinova IB, Khaspekova SG, Golubeva NV, Shustova ON, Antonova OA, Karganov MY, et al. Comparison of the size of membrane microparticles of different cellular origin by dynamic light scattering. Doklady Biochemistry and Biophysics. 2016;**470**(1):322-325

[24] Wu ZH, Ji CL, Li H, Qiu GX, Gao CJ, Weng XS. Membrane microparticles and diseases. European Review for Medical and Pharmacological Sciences. 2013;**17**(18):2420-2427

[25] Wu YW, Goubran H, Seghatchian J, Burnouf T. Smart blood cell and microvesicle-based Trojan horse drug delivery: Merging expertise in blood transfusion and biomedical engineering in the field of nanomedicine. Transfusion and Apheresis Science. 2016;**54**(2):309-318

[26] Al-Nedawi K, Meehan B, Micallef J, Lhotak V, May L, Guha A, et al. Intercellular transfer of the oncogenic receptor EGFRvIII by microvesicles derived from tumour cells. Nature Cell Biology. 2008;**10**(5):619-624

[27] Zhou W, Fong MY, Min Y, Somlo G, Liu L, Palomares MR, et al. Cancer-secreted miR-105 destroys vascular endothelial barriers to promote metastasis. Cancer Cell. 2014;**25**(4):501-515

[28] Thierry AR, El Messaoudi S, Gahan PB, Anker P, Stroun M. Origins, structures, and functions of circulating DNA in oncology. Cancer and Metastasis Reviews. 2016;**35**(3):347-376

[29] Rykova EY, Morozkin ES, Ponomaryova AA, Loseva EM, Zaporozhchenko IA, Cherdyntseva NV, et al. Cell-free and cell-bound circulating nucleic acid complexes: Mechanisms of generation, concentration and content. Expert Opinion on Biological Therapy. 2012;**12** Suppl 1(1):S141-153

[30] Yanez-Mo M, Siljander PR, Andreu Z, Zavec AB, Borras FE, Buzas EI, et al. Biological properties of extracellular vesicles and their physiological functions. Journal of Extracellular Vesicles. 2015;**4**(27066):27066

[31] Cossetti C, Smith JA, Iraci N, Leonardi T, Alfaro-Cervello C, Pluchino S. Extracellular membrane vesicles and immune regulation in the brain. Frontiers in Physiology. 2012; **3**(117):117

[32] Raposo G, Nijman HW, Stoorvogel W, Liejendekker R, Harding CV, Melief CJ, et al. B lymphocytes secrete antigen-presenting vesicles. Journal of Experimental Medicine. 1996;**183**(3):1161-1172

[33] Robbins PD, Morelli AE. Regulation of immune responses by extracellular vesicles. Nature Reviews Immunology. 2014;**14**(3):195-208

[34] Montecalvo A, Larregina AT, Shufesky WJ, Stolz DB, Sullivan ML, Karlsson JM, et al. Mechanism of transfer of functional microRNAs between mouse dendritic cells via exosomes. Blood. 2012;**119**(3):756-766

[35] Kim HK, Song KS, Park YS, Kang YH, Lee YJ, Lee KR, et al. Elevated levels of circulating platelet microparticles, VEGF, IL-6 and RANTES in patients with gastric cancer: Possible role of a metastasis predictor. European Journal of Cancer. 2003;**39**(2):184-191

[36] Ratajczak J, Wysoczynski M, Hayek F, Janowska-Wieczorek A, Ratajczak MZ. Membrane-derived microvesicles: Important and underappreciated mediators of cell-to-cell communication. Leukemia. 2006;**20**(9):1487-1495

[37] De Broe ME, Wieme RJ, Logghe GN, Roels F. Spontaneous shedding of plasma membrane fragments by human cells in vivo and in vitro. Clinica Chimica Acta. 1977;**81**(3):237-245

[38] Steffen P, Jung A, Nguyen DB, Muller T, Bernhardt I, Kaestner L, et al. Stimulation of human red blood cells leads to Ca2+-mediated intercellular adhesion. Cell Calcium. 2011;**50**(1):54-61

[39] Kaestner L, Steffen P, Nguyen DB, Wang J, Wagner-Britz L, Jung A, Wagner C, Bernhardt I. Lysophosphatidic acid induced red blood cell aggregation in vitro. Bioelectrochemistry. 2012;**87**:89-95

[40] Burnouf T, Chou ML, Goubran H, Cognasse F, Garraud O, Seghatchian J. An overview of the role of microparticles/microvesicles in blood components: Are they clinically beneficial or harmful? Transfusion and Apheresis Science. 2015;**53**(2):137-145

[41] Nguyen DB, LW-B, Maia S, Steffen P, Wagner C, Kaestner K, Bernhardt I. Regulation of phosphatidylserine exposure in red blood cells. Cellular Physiology and Biochemistry. 2011;**28**:847-856

[42] Zecher D, Cumpelik A, Schifferli JA. Erythrocyte-derived microvesicles amplify systemic inflammation by thrombin-dependent activation of complement. Arteriosclerosis Thrombosis and Vascular Biology. 2014;**34**(2):313-320

[43] Levin G, Sukhareva E, Lavrentieva A. Impact of microparticles derived from erythrocytes on fibrinolysis. Journal of Thrombosis and Thrombolysis. 2016;**41**(3):452-458

[44] Chang M, Hsiao JK, Yao M, Chien LY, Hsu SC, Ko BS, et al. Homologous RBC-derived vesicles as ultrasmall carriers of iron oxide for magnetic resonance imaging of stem cells. Nanotechnology. 2010;**21**(23):235103

[45] Mantel PY, Hjelmqvist D, Walch M, Kharoubi-Hess S, Nilsson S, Ravel D, et al. Infected erythrocyte-derived extracellular vesicles alter vascular function via regulatory Ago2-miRNA complexes in malaria. Nature Communications. 2016;**7**(12727):12727

[46] Ankarklev J, Hjelmqvist D, Mantel P-Y. Uncovering the role of Erythrocyte-Derived extracellular vesicles in malaria: From immune regulation to cell communication. Journal of Circulating Biomarkers. 2014:1-11

[47] Bosman GJ, Werre JM, Willekens FL, Novotny VM. Erythrocyte ageing in vivo and in vitro: Structural aspects and implications for transfusion. Transfusion Medicine. 2008;**18**(6):335-347

[48] Kim DK, Lee J, Simpson RJ, Lotvall J, Gho YS. EVpedia: A community web resource for prokaryotic and eukaryotic extracellular vesicles research. Seminars in Cell and Developmental Biology. 2015;**40**:4-7

[49] Devaux PF, Herrmann A, Ohlwein N, Kozlov MM. How lipid flippases can modulate membrane structure. Biochimica et Biophysica Acta. 2008;**1778**(7-8):1591-1600

[50] Bevers EM, Williamson PL. Phospholipid scramblase: An update. FEBS Letters. 2010;**584**(13):2724-2730

[51] Bevers EM, Comfurius P, Dekkers DW, Zwaal RF. Lipid translocation across the plasma membrane of mammalian cells. Biochimica et Biophysica Acta. 1999;**1439**(3):317-330

[52] Gonzalez LJ, Gibbons E, Bailey RW, Fairbourn J, Nguyen T, Smith SK, et al. The influence of membrane physical properties on microvesicle release in human erythrocytes. PMC Biophysics. 2009;**2**(1):7

[53] Daleke DL. Regulation of phospholipid asymmetry in the erythrocyte membrane. Current Opinion in Hematology. 2008;**15**(3):191-195

[54] Daleke DL. Regulation of transbilayer plasma membrane phospholipid asymmetry. Journal of Lipid Research. 2003;**44**(2):233-242

[55] Pasini EM, Kirkegaard M, Mortensen P, Lutz HU, Thomas AW, Mann M. In-depth analysis of the membrane and cytosolic proteome of red blood cells. Blood. 2006;**108**(3):791-801

[56] Chung SM, Bae ON, Lim KM, Noh JY, Lee MY, Jung YS, et al. Lysophosphatidic acid induces thrombogenic activity through phosphatidylserine exposure and procoagulant microvesicle generation in human erythrocytes. Arteriosclerosis Thrombosis and Vascular Biology. 2007;**27**(2):414-421

[57] Williamson P, Kulick A, Zachowski A, Schlegel RA, Devaux PF. Ca2+ induces transbilayer redistribution of all major phospholipids in human erythrocytes. Biochemistry. 1992;**31**(27):6355-6360

[58] Dekkers DW, Comfurius P, Vuist WM, Billheimer JT, Dicker I, Weiss HJ, et al. Impaired Ca2+-induced tyrosine phosphorylation and defective lipid scrambling in erythrocytes from a patient with Scott syndrome: A study using an inhibitor for scramblase that mimics the defect in Scott syndrome. Blood. 1998;**91**(6):2133-2138

[59] Suzuki J, Umeda M, Sims PJ, Nagata S. Calcium-dependent phospholipid scrambling by TMEM16F. Nature. 2010;**468**(7325):834-838

[60] Kalra H, Drummen GP, Mathivanan S. Focus on extracellular vesicles: Introducing the next small big thing. International Journal of Molecular Sciences. 2016;**17**(2):170

[61] Wesseling MC, Wagner-Britz L, Nguyen DB, Asanidze S, Mutua J, Mohamed N, et al. Novel Insights in the regulation of phosphatidylserine exposure in human red blood cells. Cellular Physiology and Biochemistry. 2016;**39**(5):1941-1954

[62] Stowell SR, Smith NH, Zimring JC, Fu X, Palmer AF, Fontes J, et al. Addition of ascorbic acid solution to stored murine red blood cells increases posttransfusion recovery and decreases microparticles and alloimmunization. Transfusion. 2013;**53**(10):2248-2257

[63] Kalra H, Simpson RJ, Ji H, Aikawa E, Altevogt P, Askenase P, et al. Vesiclepedia: A compendium for extracellular vesicles with continuous community annotation. PLOS Biology. 2012;**10**(12):e1001450

[64] Kim DK, Kang B, Kim OY, Choi DS, Lee J, Kim SR, et al. EVpedia: An integrated database of high-throughput data for systemic analyses of extracellular vesicles. Journal of Extracellular Vesicles. 2013;**2**(2)

[65] Iraci N, Leonardi T, Gessler F, Vega B, Pluchino S. Focus on extracellular vesicles: Physiological role and signalling properties of extracellular membrane vesicles. International Journal of Molecular Sciences. 2016;**17**(2):171

[66] Simons M, Raposo G. Exosomes--vesicular carriers for intercellular communication. Current Opinion in Cell Biology. 2009;**21**(4):575-581

[67] Chen SY, Wang Y, Telen MJ, Chi JT. The genomic analysis of erythrocyte microRNA expression in sickle cell diseases. PLoS One. 2008;**3**(6):e2360

[68] Kina T, Ikuta K, Takayama E, Wada K, Majumdar AS, Weissman IL, et al. The monoclonal antibody TER-119 recognizes a molecule associated with glycophorin A and specifically marks the late stages of murine erythroid lineage. British Journal of Haematology. 2000;**109**(2):280-287

[69] Burnier L, Fontana P, Kwak BR, Angelillo-Scherrer A. Cell-derived microparticles in haemostasis and vascular medicine. Thrombosis and Haemostasis. 2009;**101**(3):439-451

[70] Wubbolts R, Leckie RS, Veenhuizen PT, Schwarzmann G, Mobius W, Hoernschemeyer J, et al. Proteomic and biochemical analyses of human B cell-derived exosomes. Potential implications for their function and multivesicular body formation. Journal of Biological Chemistry. 2003;**278**(13):10963-10972

[71] Oldenborg PA, Zheleznyak A, Fang YF, Lagenaur CF, Gresham HD, Lindberg FP. Role of CD47 as a marker of self on red blood cells. Science. 2000;**288**(5473):2051-2054

[72] Ishikawa-Sekigami T, Kaneko Y, Okazawa H, Tomizawa T, Okajo J, Saito Y, et al. SHPS-1 promotes the survival of circulating erythrocytes through inhibition of phagocytosis by splenic macrophages. Blood. 2006;**107**(1):341-348

[73] Burger P, Hilarius-Stokman P, de Korte D, van den Berg TK, van Bruggen R. CD47 functions as a molecular switch for erythrocyte phagocytosis. Blood. 2012;**119**(23):5512-5521

[74] Villa CH, Pan DC, Zaitsev S, Cines DB, Siegel DL, Muzykantov VR. Delivery of drugs bound to erythrocytes: New avenues for an old intravascular carrier. Therapeutic Delivery. 2015;**6**(7):795-826

[75] Muzykantov VR. Drug delivery by red blood cells: Vascular carriers designed by mother nature. Expert Opinion on Drug Delivery. 2010;**7**(4):403-427

[76] Burger P, de Korte D, van den Berg TK, van Bruggen R. CD47 in Erythrocyte ageing and clearance - the dutch point of view. Transfusion Medicine and Hemotherapy. 2012; **39**(5):348-352

[77] Per-Arne O. Role of CD47 and signal regulatory protein alpha (SIRPalpha) in regulating the clearance of viable or aged blood cells. Transfusion Medicine and Hemotherapy. 2012;**39**(5):315-320

[78] Bosman GJ, Willekens FL, Werre JM. Erythrocyte aging: A more than superficial resemblance to apoptosis? Cellular Physiology and Biochemistry. 2005;**16**(1-3):1-8

[79] Bosman GJ, Lasonder E, Groenen-Dopp YA, Willekens FL, Werre JM. The proteome of erythrocyte-derived microparticles from plasma: New clues for erythrocyte aging and vesiculation. Journal of Proteomics. 2012;**76**:Spec No.:203-10

[80] Bosman GJ, Lasonder E, Groenen-Dopp YA, Willekens FL, Werre JM, Novotny VM. Comparative proteomics of erythrocyte aging in vivo and in vitro. Journal of Proteomics. 2010;**73**(3):396-402

[81] Iida K, Whitlow MB, Nussenzweig V. Membrane vesiculation protects erythrocytes from destruction by complement. Journal of Immunology. 1991;**147**(8):2638-2642

[82] Kriebardis AG, Antonelou MH, Stamoulis KE, Economou-Petersen E, Margaritis LH, Papassideri IS. RBC-derived vesicles during storage: Ultrastructure, protein composition, oxidation, and signaling components. Transfusion. 2008;**48**(9):1943-1953

[83] Prudent M, Crettaz D, Delobel J, Seghatchian J, Tissot JD, Lion N. Differences between calcium-stimulated and storage-induced erythrocyte-derived microvesicles. Transfusion and Apheresis Science. 2015;**53**(2):153-158

[84] Piccin A, Van Schilfgaarde M, Smith O. The importance of studying red blood cells microparticles. Journal of Blood Transfusion. 2015;**13**(2):172-173

[85] Menck K, Bleckmann A, Schulz M, Ries L, Binder C. Isolation and characterization of microvesicles from peripheral blood. Journal of Visualized Experiments. 2017;**6**(119): 55057

[86] Jayachandran M, Miller VM, Heit JA, Owen WG. Methodology for isolation, identification and characterization of microvesicles in peripheral blood. Journal of Immunology Methods. 2012;**375**(1-2):207-214

[87] Kong F, Zhang L, Wang H, Yuan G, Guo A, Li Q, et al. Impact of collection, isolation and storage methodology of circulating microvesicles on flow cytometric analysis. Experimental and Therapeutic Medicine. 2015;**10**(6):2093-2101

[88] Lee M, Ban J-J, Im W, Kim M. Influence of storage condition on exosome recovery. Biotechnology and Bioprocess Engineering. 2016;**21**(2):299-304

[89] Zhou H, Yuen PS, Pisitkun T, Gonzales PA, Yasuda H, Dear JW, et al. Collection, storage, preservation, and normalization of human urinary exosomes for biomarker discovery. Kidney International. 2006;**69**(8):1471-1476

[90] Wisgrill L, Lamm C, Hartmann J, Preissing F, Dragosits K, Bee A, et al. Peripheral blood microvesicles secretion is influenced by storage time, temperature, and anticoagulants. Cytometry Part A. 2016;**89**(7):663-672

[91] Lotvall J, Hill AF, Hochberg F, Buzas EI, Di Vizio D, Gardiner C, et al. Minimal experimental requirements for definition of extracellular vesicles and their functions: A position statement from the International Society for Extracellular Vesicles. Journal of Extracellular Vesicles. 2014;**3**(26913):26913

[92] Nordin JZ, Lee Y, Vader P, Mager I, Johansson HJ, Heusermann W, et al. Ultrafiltration with size-exclusion liquid chromatography for high yield isolation of extracellular vesicles preserving intact biophysical and functional properties. Nanomedicine. 2015;**11**(4):879-883

[93] Lener T, Gimona M, Aigner L, Borger V, Buzas E, Camussi G, et al. Applying extracellular vesicles based therapeutics in clinical trials - an ISEV position paper. Journal of Extracellular Vesicles. 2015;**4**(30087):30087

[94] Lorincz AM, Timar CI, Marosvari KA, Veres DS, Otrokocsi L, Kittel A, et al. Effect of storage on physical and functional properties of extracellular vesicles derived from neutrophilic granulocytes. Journal of Extracellular Vesicles. 2014;**3**(25465):25465

[95] Lamparski HG, Metha-Damani A, Yao JY, Patel S, Hsu DH, Ruegg C, et al. Production and characterization of clinical grade exosomes derived from dendritic cells. Journal of Immunology Methods. 2002;**270**(2):211-226

[96] Grisendi G, Finetti E, Manganaro D, Cordova N, Montagnani G, Spano C, et al. Detection of microparticles from human red blood cells by multiparametric flow cytometry. Journal of Blood Transfusion. 2015;**13**(2):274-280

[97] Alvarez-Erviti L, Seow Y, Yin H, Betts C, Lakhal S, Wood MJ. Delivery of siRNA to the mouse brain by systemic injection of targeted exosomes. Nature Biotechnology. 2011;**29**(4):341-345

[98] Godbey DABaW. Liposomes for use in gene delivery. Journal of Drug Delivery. 2011;**2011**(Article ID 326497):12. DOI: 0.1155/2011/326497

[99] van der Meel R, Fens MH, Vader P, van Solinge WW, Eniola-Adefeso O, Schiffelers RM. Extracellular vesicles as drug delivery systems: Lessons from the liposome field. Journal of Controlled Release. 2014;**195**:72-85

[100] Kotmakci M, Bozok Cetintas V. Extracellular vesicles as natural nanosized delivery systems for Small-Molecule drugs and genetic material: Steps towards the future nanomedicines. Journal of Pharmacy & Pharmaceutical Sciences. **2015**;18(3):396-413

[101] Yuan A, Farber EL, Rapoport AL, Tejada D, Deniskin R, Akhmedov NB, et al. Transfer of microRNAs by embryonic stem cell microvesicles. PLoS One. 2009;**4**(3):e4722

[102] van Dommelen SM, Vader P, Lakhal S, Kooijmans SA, van Solinge WW, Wood MJ, et al. Microvesicles and exosomes: Opportunities for cell-derived membrane vesicles in drug delivery. Journal of Controlled Release. 2012;**161**(2):635-644

[103] Tian Y, Li S, Song J, Ji T, Zhu M, Anderson GJ, et al. A doxorubicin delivery platform using engineered natural membrane vesicle exosomes for targeted tumor therapy. Biomaterials. 2014;**35**(7):2383-2390

[104] Sun D, Zhuang X, Xiang X, Liu Y, Zhang S, Liu C, et al. A novel nanoparticle drug delivery system: The anti-inflammatory activity of curcumin is enhanced when encapsulated in exosomes. Molecular Therapy. 2010;**18**(9):1606-1614

[105] Zhang L, Valencia CA, Dong B, Chen M, Guan PJ, Pan L. Transfer of microRNAs by extracellular membrane microvesicles: A nascent crosstalk model in tumor pathogenesis, especially tumor cell-microenvironment interactions. Journal of Hematology & Oncology. 2015;**8**(14):14

[106] Becker A, Thakur BK, Weiss JM, Kim HS, Peinado H, Lyden D. Extracellular vesicles in cancer: Cell-to-Cell mediators of metastasis. Cancer Cell. 2016;**30**(6):836-848

[107] Pultz BD, da Luz FA, Faria SS, de Souza LP, Brigido Tavares PC, Goulart VA, et al. The multifaceted role of extracellular vesicles in metastasis: Priming the soil for seeding. International Journal of Cancer. 2017;**16**(10):30595

[108] Li J, Zhang Y, Liu Y, Dai X, Li W, Cai X, et al. Microvesicle-mediated transfer of microRNA-150 from monocytes to endothelial cells promotes angiogenesis. Journal of Biological Chemistry. 2013;**288**(32):23586-23596

[109] Liang H, Yan X, Pan Y, Wang Y, Wang N, Li L, et al. MicroRNA-223 delivered by platelet-derived microvesicles promotes lung cancer cell invasion via targeting tumor suppressor EPB41L3. Molecular Cancer. 2015;**14**(58):58

[110] Zhang Y, Li L, Yu J, Zhu D, Zhang Y, Li X, et al. Microvesicle-mediated delivery of transforming growth factor beta1 siRNA for the suppression of tumor growth in mice. Biomaterials. 2014;**35**(14):4390-4400

[111] Lamichhane TN, Raiker RS, Jay SM. Exogenous DNA Loading into extracellular vesicles via electroporation is Size-Dependent and enables limited gene delivery. Molecular Pharmaceutics. 2015;**12**(10):3650-3657

[112] Waldenstrom A, Genneback N, Hellman U, Ronquist G. Cardiomyocyte microvesicles contain DNA/RNA and convey biological messages to target cells. PLoS One. 2012;**7**(4):e34653

[113] Mizrak A, Bolukbasi MF, Ozdener GB, Brenner GJ, Madlener S, Erkan EP, et al. Genetically engineered microvesicles carrying suicide mRNA/protein inhibit schwannoma tumor growth. Molecular Therapy. 2013;**21**(1):101-108

[114] Lakhal S, Wood MJ. Exosome nanotechnology: An emerging paradigm shift in drug delivery: Exploitation of exosome nanovesicles for systemic in vivo delivery of RNAi heralds new horizons for drug delivery across biological barriers. Bioessays. 2011;**33**(10):737-741

[115] Kooijmans SA, Vader P, van Dommelen SM, van Solinge WW, Schiffelers RM. Exosome mimetics: A novel class of drug delivery systems. International Journal of Nanomedicine. 2012;**7**:1525-1541

[116] Chaput N, Flament C, Viaud S, Taieb J, Roux S, Spatz A, et al. Dendritic cell derived-exosomes: Biology and clinical implementations. Journal of Leukocyte Biology. 2006;**80**(3):471-478

[117] Johnsen KB, Gudbergsson JM, Skov MN, Pilgaard L, Moos T, Duroux M. A comprehensive overview of exosomes as drug delivery vehicles - endogenous nanocarriers for targeted cancer therapy. Biochimica et Biophysica Acta. 2014;**1846**(1):75-87

[118] Vader P, Kooijmans SA, Stremersch S, Raemdonck K. New considerations in the preparation of nucleic acid-loaded extracellular vesicles. Therapeutic Delivery. 2014; **5**(2):105-107

[119] Kosaka N, Iguchi H, Yoshioka Y, Takeshita F, Matsuki Y, Ochiya T. Secretory mechanisms and intercellular transfer of microRNAs in living cells. Journal of Biological Chemistry. 2010;**285**(23):17442-17452

[120] Ohno S, Takanashi M, Sudo K, Ueda S, Ishikawa A, Matsuyama N, et al. Systemically injected exosomes targeted to EGFR deliver antitumor microRNA to breast cancer cells. Molecular Therapy. 2013;**21**(1):185-191

[121] Zhou Y, Xiong M, Fang L, Jiang L, Wen P, Dai C, et al. miR-21-containing microvesicles from injured tubular epithelial cells promote tubular phenotype transition by targeting PTEN protein. The American Journal of Pathology. 2013;**183**(4):1183-1196

[122] Wahlgren J, De LKT, Brisslert M, Vaziri Sani F, Telemo E, Sunnerhagen P, et al. Plasma exosomes can deliver exogenous short interfering RNA to monocytes and lymphocytes. Nucleic Acids Research. 2012;**40**(17):e130

Chapter 8

Exosome Isolation: Is There an Optimal Method with Regard to Diagnosis or Treatment?

Mustafa Kotmakçı and Gülşah Erel Akbaba

Additional information is available at the end of the chapter

http://dx.doi.org/10.5772/intechopen.69407

Abstract

Extracellular vesicles (EV) gained considerable interest in recent years as both diagnostic tools and templates for therapeutic applications. EVs carry a number of cell-specific markers which gave researchers the opportunity of employing them as liquid biopsies causing no discomfort to patients. On the other hand, they are very exciting candidates for drug delivery due to their eobiotic origin, physicochemical and size characteristics. Isolation of EVs is performed by several strategies, having advantages and disatvantages over each other. As such, the method of EV isolation and in particular exosome isolation determines the quality and purity of obtained vesicles. In this chapter, extracellular vesicle isolation methods are evaluated with regard to their further use. Methods such as ultracentrifugation with different modifications, size exclusion chromatography, ultrafiltration, affinity and precipitation are compared with respect to the yield efficacy and purity of isolates. Furthermore, the advantages and disadvantages of different methods according to the purpose of use are revealed. Recent progress and remaining challenges in the isolation of EVs with regard to diagnosis and treatment is reviewed and discussed. In order to select the most suitable method researchers should clearly define purity, yield, quantity and quality requirements for exosomes, and consider disadvantages of distinct isolation methods.

Keywords: exosomes, extracellular vesicles, ultracentrifugation, size exclusion chromatography, precipitation, ultrafiltration, affinity isolation

1. Introduction

Extracellular vesicles (EVs) are nano-sized membrane vesicles, released by almost every cell types. EVs are shown to play crucial roles in many physiological events, as well as many pathological processes. In the past decade, extensive research has been done using exosomes as vehicles for diagnostic and therapeutic application. Previous studies showed that exosomes are promising systems for drug and nucleic acid delivery. Also, they might be promising tools for diagnosis. Different types of EVs, including exosomes, microvesicles and apoptotic bodies are released by cells. The vesicles are diverse and their quantity and quality depend on the type and origin of the cells. Among these, exosomes are the smallest vesicle type, with sizes ranging from 30 to 120 nm. They originate from multivesicular bodies (MVBs), the form of endosomes at a later stage of maturation. Exosomes are formed by inward budding of the endosomal membrane and accumulate in these MVBs. Later, these small vesicles in MVBs are released from the cells upon fusion of MVBs with the plasma membrane [1, 2]. In contrast, microvesicles (MVs) are larger (50 nm–1 μm) and more heterogeneous in size. MVs are formed through direct outward budding of the plasma membrane. A heterogeneous population of vesicles (50 nm–5 μm) which are named apoptotic bodies are released during late stages of the programmed cell death. Each EV subtype contains different amounts of cargo molecules the identity of which is more or less similar among EV subtypes [3].

In different applications, it is important to make a clear distinction between MVs and exosomes because of the fact that they are different both in protein and genetic material content, and in size characteristics. This is important when post-purification processes such as protein characterization/isolation, RNA sequencing, targeted or conventional application in therapeutics delivery are to be investigated. This issue is still scarcely addressed and more research is needed in order to develop specific isolation methods for different EV subtypes. Also, there is still not enough knowledge about how the isolation methods affect physicochemical properties of exosomes. As can be seen from their size distribution and similarities between their cargo molecules, there is no strict border separating different EV subtypes. As the result, it is difficult to obtain highly purified exosome isolates that are completely devoid of other EV types. Given the fact that more and more research focuses on the potential of EVs for diagnostic and therapeutic application, the need of a reproducible method for their purification becomes more prominent.

Due to the complex nature of both intracellular matrix and extracellular environment from which EVs are isolated, not only the desired structures are attained. From biological fluids, contaminants such as proteins, lipoproteins and nucleic acids are also isolated together with the EVs [4–6]. Isolates from cell culture media are contaminated by supplements such as antibiotics and extraneous proteins and EVs coming from fetal bovine serum (FBS) [5, 7]. Prokaryotic contamination is also reported for body fluid EV preparations [8]. All of these contaminants affect the downstream applications of EVs.

In diagnostic applications, these contaminants could lead to false-positive results and subsequently erroneous interpretations. For example, free proteins can lead to over-estimation of the protein cargo of EVs, and, if the protein concentration is considered for normalization of samples, this could lead to significant inconsistencies between results of different research groups.

In order to circumvent any potential interference with the therapeutic efficacy of the active compound, and to minimize the risk of unpredicted side effects, the composition simplicity of drug delivery systems is of utmost importance. Even though there are small number of ingredients in conventional nanoparticle-based drug delivery systems (liposomes, solid

http://dx.doi.org/10.5772/intechopen.69407

lipid nanoparticles, polymeric nanoparticles, etc.), there are still many debated aspects related to their safety. Considering their nature, EVs are obviously much more complicated than conventional nanoparticulate therapeutics. Therefore, in the therapeutic application field, impurities in EV isolates can be much more confusing. When EVs are isolated from cells designed to express a particular RNA molecule, other changes could also occur in the cellular machinery, and as a consequence, these could contribute to loading of unknown impurities into the EV lumen, leading to false-positive results or even toxicity [9]. This problem can be accomplished, at least in part, by optimizing the isolation protocols, applying extra purification steps and by investigation of sensitive detection techniques for biomolecules [10–14]. However, currently, there is still not single method which ensures EV isolation fully devoid of impurities. In this respect, different isolation methods will be discussed for their applicability in isolation of exosomes intended either for diagnostic or therapeutic purposes.

2. Isolation methods and their convenience in different applications

EVs can be isolated from different types of bodily fluids such as blood, urine and saliva. Depending on the source cell, EVs took part in different roles in the body ecosystem and they are able to overcome natural barriers as cellular membrane, blood-brain barrier and escape the immune system, etc. [1]. Moreover, their immunologic and cytotoxic activities are very low. Despite EVs' promise for diagnostic and therapeutic applications, effective and pure isolation is still a problem which should be overcome. Existing isolation methods cause difficulty in terms of purity and reproducibility [15]. Besides, in some applications, it is important to make a clear distinction between MVs and exosomes because of the fact that they are different both in protein and genetic material content, and in size characteristics. This is important when post-purification processes such as protein characterization/isolation, RNA sequencing, targeted or conventional application in therapeutics delivery are to be investigated, as each EV subtype contains different amounts of cargo molecules [3]. This issue is still scarcely addressed and more research is needed in order to develop specific isolation methods for different EV subtypes.

Based on the main principle employed in the isolation process, there are basically five EV isolation methods. These are (1) Centrifugation-based methods, (2) Chromatography-based isolation, (3) Precipitation-based isolation, (4) Filtration-based isolation and (5) Affinity-based isolation. Each of these methods can be applied either individually or in combination with others in order to achieve higher yield or purity. **Table 1** summarizes the methods for EV isolation.

2.1. Centrifugation-based EV isolation

Owing to their colloidal size, EVs tend to sediment only under high centrifugal forces. The classical method for EV isolation is differential ultracentrifugation, as used in early exosome studies [16]. While this isolation method is still the most widely used approach, often with modifications of the duration, conditions and the speed of centrifugation steps, several subtechniques have since been developed. Two commonly used techniques based on centrifugation are differential ultracentrifugation and density gradient ultracentrifugation.

Isolation method	Principle	Required instrumentation and consumables
• Differential centrifugation	• Sedimentation under high centrifugal forces based on density and particle size	General purpose centrifuge, ultracentrifuge, conical centrifuge tubes, ultracentrifuge tubes
• Density gradient ultracentrifugation	• Separation of EVs and other non-vesicular components based on their buoyant density in a density gradient under high centrifugal forces	
• Chromatography-based isolation	• Size exclusion chromatography or gel filtration chromatography. Separation is achieved due to penetration of smaller particles into the pores of a matrix material during elution through a column	Prefilled or custom made chromatography columns, matrix material
• Ultrafiltration	• Separation of EV subtypes and proteins using membrane filters. Separation is based on the size of different particles	Ultrafiltration device equipped with peristaltic pump, ultrafiltration cartridges, centrifugal filtration cartridges
• Polymer-based precipitation	• Reduction of EVs' aqueous solubility in the presence of PEG	General purpose centrifuge, conical centrifuge tubes
• Salt precipitation	• Charge neutralization by adding salt solution followed by reduction of EV solubility in low pH	
• Charge-based precipitation	• Enhanced precipitation of EVs by addition of protamine sulphate based on their negative surface charge	
• Affinity purification (specific antibodies, lectins and heparin)	• Capturing different EVs owing to specific molecules present on their membranes	Antibody coated chromatography matrices, microfluidic devices

Table 1. Commonly used EV isolation methods.

3. Differential ultracentrifugation

This method generally employs at least one step of low-speed (2000 g) centrifugation. In this step, whole cells and cell debris such as apoptotic bodies are removed. A second step of centrifugation at higher g-force (5000–10,000 g) ensures removal of large EV aggregates and protein aggregates. The supernatant is then subjected to 1–3 h ultracentrifugation (≥100,000 g) at 4°C. EVs and high-density proteins are enriched at the bottom of the ultracentrifuge tube in form of a tiny, barely visible sediment. The supernatant containing small proteins, cell culture supplements, buffer ions etc. is carefully discarded and the pellet is washed by adding cold phosphate buffered saline (PBS) and dispersing by vigorous vortexing or pipetting. A second step of ultracentrifugation is performed. The supernatant is discarded, and finally, washed EVs are collected in little amount of cold PBS. The general steps of differential ultracentrifugation method for EV isolation are presented in **Figure 1**.

Materials required for this isolation method are sterile conical centrifuge tubes, clean and sterile ultracentrifuge tubes, pipettes for handling the liquid material, PBS or other suitable buffer according to the downstream applications. Equipment for the procedure includes conventional benchtop centrifuge with cooling mode; ultracentrifuge capable of performing centrifugation at g-forces higher than 100,000 g; a laminar flow biosafety hood in order to provide aseptic working conditions, especially when EVs are going to be used as therapeutic delivery systems.

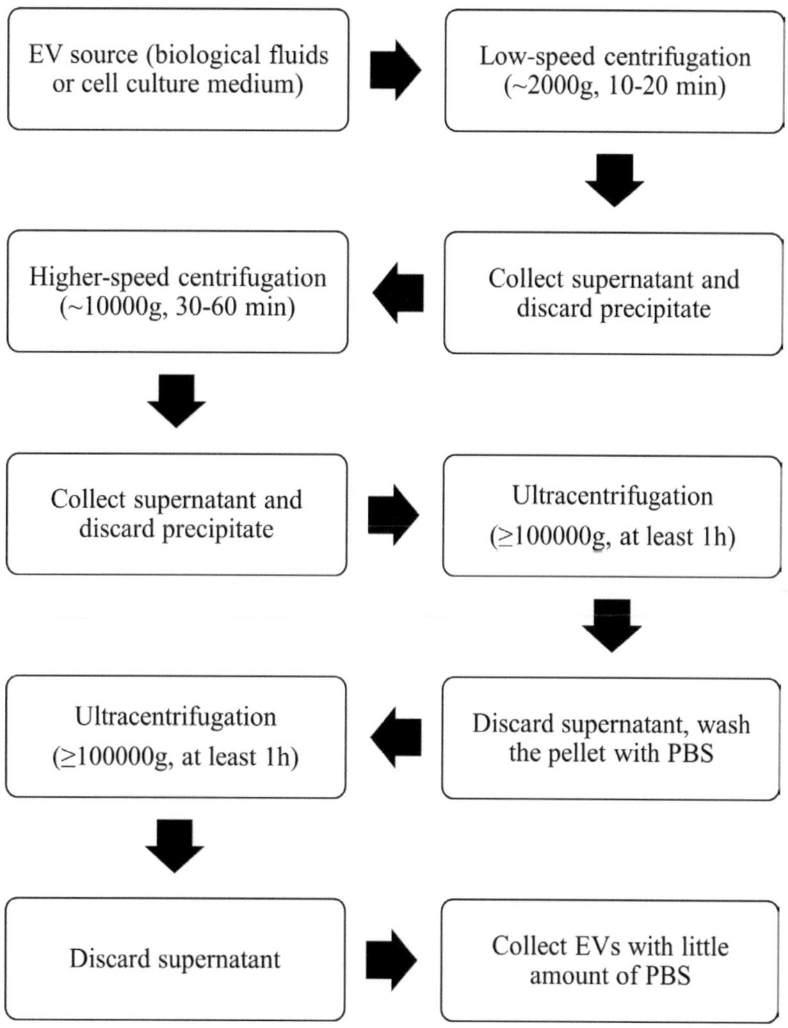

Figure 1. General steps followed during EV isolation by differential ultracentrifugation. In this method, the source of EVs is first cleared from cells and cell debris by performing two steps of centrifugation in a conventional benchtop centrifuge. Afterwards, the cleared supernatant is ultracentrifuged at >100,000× g for at least 1 h, washed with PBS, ultracentrifuged again, and finally, the EVs are collected from the ultracentifuge tubes.

The limitations of this method are its time-consuming protocol and possibility of aggregations under high centrifugal forces [15]. Lamparski et al. performed a comprehensive study on the development of clinical grade, good manufacturing practice (GMP)-compliant method for exosome purification [17]. They compared differential ultracentrifugation, ultrafiltration-cushion ultracentrifugation methods. The method of differential centrifugation produced highly variable results for exosome yield. Ultrafiltration followed by cushion ultracentrifugation has given more stable exosome yield with higher recovery, and regulatory compliance [17].

Tauro et al. investigated ultracentrifugation, density gradient separation and immunoaffinity capture methods [18]. Exosomes were isolated from 500 µl cell culture supernatant and the yield of applied methods were analysed. In this set of experiments, ultracentrifugation has given the best yield (375 µg), followed by density gradient separation (150 µg) and immunoaffinity capture (195 µg). The size uniformity of exosomes has been shown to alter according to the isolation method. In this study, the immunoprecipitation method has been considered the best for exosome capture, as it yielded exosomes that have greater homogeneity and higher exosome-associated protein content [18].

4. Density gradient ultracentrifugation

In density gradient ultracentrifugation, almost the same steps are followed as in differential ultracentrifugation. Materials required for this isolation method are sterile conical centrifuge tubes, clean and sterile ultracentrifuge tubes, pipettes for handling the liquid material, sucrose or iodixanol for preparation of discontinuous gradient, PBS or other suitable buffer according to the downstream applications [19]. Equipments required for performing this procedure are the same as those described in differential ultracentrifugation method.

The EVs are first isolated by applying the differential centrifugation steps and the first ultracentrifugation step, as described under the differential ultracentrifugation, or alternatively, the isolation medium is concentrated using centrifugal filters. Next, a discontinuous sucrose or iodixanol gradient is prepared in ultracentrifugation tubes. For this purpose, sucrose solutions of gradually decreasing concentration are overlaid atop of each other. Crude EV pellet or concentrated isolation medium is then resuspended in little amount of PBS or buffer of choice, loaded on the gradient liquid and ultracentrifuged for extended period of time in order to separate EVs based on their buoyant density in the discontinuous viscous fluid [14, 18, 20]. The general steps of density gradient ultracentrifugation method for EV isolation are presented in **Figure 2**.

The ultracentrifugation method remains the most widely used approach for EV isolation. Lack of technical information about the type and the diameter of the rotor used, the volume and viscosity of the sample all represent challenges for establishing a standardized ultracentrifugation-based method [21].

The limitation of density gradient ultracentrifugation is its even long-lasting ultracentrifugation step as compared to differential ultracentrifugation. Moreover, this method requires an

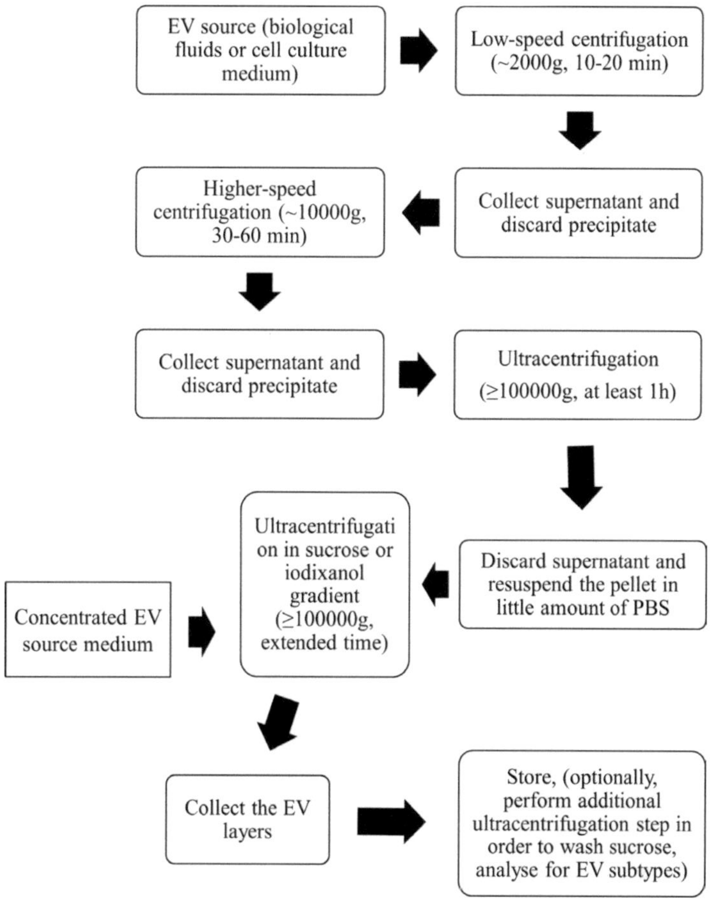

Figure 2. General steps followed during EV isolation by density gradient ultracentrifugation. This method is similar to differential ultracentrifugation to the first ultracentrifuge step. The collected EVs are then transferred on top of a gradient-forming agent and ultracentrifuged for extended period of time. EVs are separated as individual layers owing to the differences in their buoyant density and particle size. Finally, EVs are collected and analysed.

additional wash step in order to remove the density gradient-forming agent. On the other hand, its primary advantage is that several layers can be drawn after density gradient ultracentrifugation and each of these layers can be characterized in order to distinguish between different EV subtypes separated owing to their buoyant density.

4.1. Chromatography-based EV isolation

Size exclusion chromatography (SEC), also known as gel filtration chromatography, employs size difference of exosomes, microvesicles, apoptotic bodies, proteins and other components present in biological materials. The source material for EV isolation is loaded on a column prefilled with a stationary phase such as Sepharose© and Sephacryl©. A mobile phase, usually phosphate buffered saline, is then allowed to pass through the column. While the mobile phase passes through the column, it draws EVs into the stationary phase. During this process, smaller molecules such as proteins and small vesicles—the exosomes interact with the pores of the stationary phase, leading to relative deceleration of their movement speed as compared with that of larger structures. As the result, EV subtypes are separated from each other as individual populations. Generally, these particle populations are collected in small fractions and each fraction is then analysed in terms of particle size and specific markers. Suitable fractions are then pooled and used for further downstream applications. General steps followed during SEC purification of EVs are schematized in **Figure 3**. Equipments required for isolation of exosomes by SEC are a prefilled column and a mobile phase to perform the elution (usually PBS). Fractions are collected in microcentrifuge tubes for later analysis and downstream applications. Alternatively, the SEC columns can be custom-designed for investigational purposes—a syringe with removed plunger, or a small-volume burette could perform well as an empty column to be filled with a suitable chromatography resin of researchers' choice.

An efficient single step EV isolation based on chromatography is described by Böing et al. [12]. They used Sepharose CL-2B to create a separate column for size exclusion chromatography. As compared to the ultracentrifugation method from the literature, having highly varying EV yields (2–80 %), this method was superior with 43% stable recovery of EVs, and almost complete removal of contaminating proteins. Furthermore, the method takes as little time as less than 20 minutes to complete [12]. Disadvantages of this method are (1) the accessibility of the chromatography column to contamination, therefore aseptic working conditions should be ensured especially if the isolated EVs are intended for therapeutic use; (2) a large number of fractions should be collected and analysed in order to make sure complete separation of EV subtypes and contaminating proteins and (3) contrarily to the simplicity and time effectiveness of the separation protocol, post-isolation analysis of each fraction may be quite time consuming.

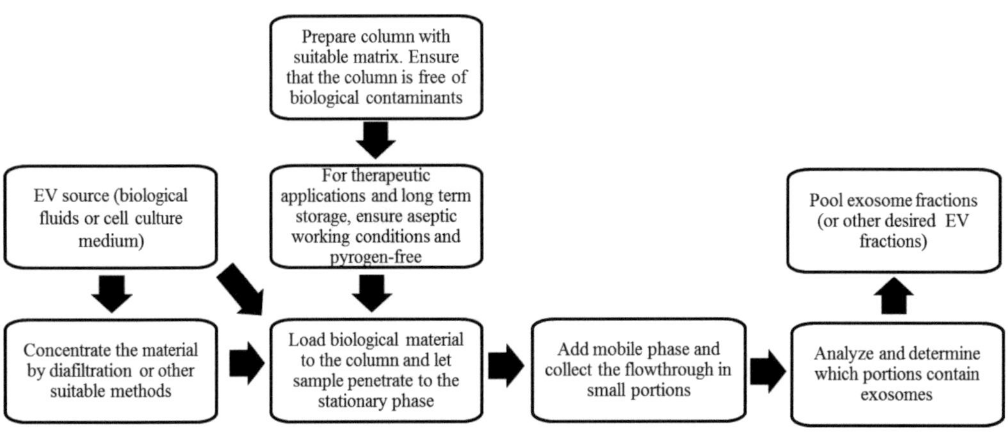

Figure 3. General steps followed during EV isolation by size exclusion chromatography. EV source is either directly loaded to the column, or first concentrated by a suitable method in order to increase the yield and then loaded to the column. Subsequently, the mobile phase is added and gravity-driven elution is performed.

4.2. Filtration-based EV isolation

Filtration-based isolation of EVs relies on separation of different EV subtypes from each other and from contaminating proteins due to their size. A series of filtrations is performed and cell debris, microvesicles, exosomes and free proteins are efficiently separated by this method. General steps of the filtration procedure can be seen in **Figure 4**. Required equipments for this method are: a peristaltic pump to circulate the EV suspension during the process, filtration cartridges in order to perform the separation, a sample chamber and a filtrate collection chamber. A proof-of-concept study describing the use of tangential flow filtration method for exosome isolation is performed by Heinemann et al. [22]. Authors made clear distinction between exosome and other EVs vesicles and aimed to efficiently separate them. Vesicles with much greater poly-dispersity are obtained as compared with differential filtration method. It was concluded that this method produces exosomal preparations with very high purity [22]. This method may be considered superior to ultracentrifugation method especially in cases where specific features of only exosomal fraction of extracellular vesicles are to be investigated, or if only exosomal fraction is desired for use in therapeutic delivery studies.

4.3. Precipitation-based EV isolation

A common and easy to handle way of isolating EVs is precipitation. In precipitation protocols, polymers such as polyethylene glycol (PEG) [7, 23, 24] or salt solutions such as sodium acetate [25] are used for isolation. In this method, the sample is first incubated with the precipitating agent. During incubation, the polymers reduce EVs' solubility and lead to their precipitation. After precipitation is completed, the pellet is simply collected by low-speed centrifugation. Later, it was observed that EV yield increases when the precipitation with polymer is performed in acidic pH [26]. Another approach may be precipitation of the solubilized proteins, leaving a supernatant enriched with extracellular vesicles. This method is called 'Protein Organic Solvent Precipitation (abbreviated as PROSPR)'. Acetone chloroform and trichloroacetic acid are used to precipitate proteins. After proteins are removed, EVs are concentrated by filtration or vacuum-dried for proteomic analysis [27]. More recently, charge-based precipitation of EVs has been reported. Researchers hypothesized that negatively charged EVs could interact with positively charged protamine sulphate. It was shown that charge-based precipitation in conjunction with polymer gives higher yield as compared with PEG-precipitation and

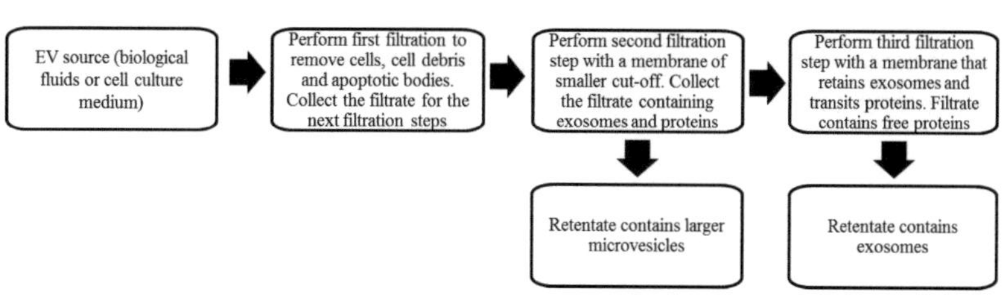

Figure 4. General steps followed during EV isolation by filtration. In this method, the source of EVs is sequentially passed through filtration cartridges with narrowing pore size. In the first step, cells and cell debris are removed. In the second filtration cartridge, the membrane passes exosomes and proteins into the filtrate while retaining microvesicles. Finally, the filtrate is passed through a cartridge with smallest pore size which passes free proteins and retains exosomes.

ultracentrifugation [23]. General steps followed during EV isolation by precipitation methods are represented in **Figure 5**. A salting-out procedure for exosome precipitation is proposed by Brownlee et al. [25]. This method employed addition of acetate ions to EV source followed by immediate precipitation of EVs due to charge neutralization. They compared the exosomes obtained with this method to these obtained by ultracentrifugation and showed that exosomes isolated by these methods are indistinguishable in respect to their size and shape characteristics. In precipitation methods, the necessary equipments are: suitable tubes for performing the precipitation, a precipitating agent of choice (polymers, electrolytes or organic solvents), buffers for performing the washes and a benchtop centrifuge to collect the formed precipitate.

4.4. Affinity-based EV isolation

Perhaps the most promising method for specific exosome isolation is the affinity precipitation in which specific antibodies are used. The most commonly employed antibodies in this method are monoclonal antibodies against specific exosomal membrane proteins (CD63, CD81, CD82, CD9, EpCam and Rab5). These antibodies are used alone or in combination [2]. Practically, the antibodies could be fixed on different types of materials such as magnetic beads [19, 28] or microfluidic devices [29–31]. The isolation is based on the binding efficiency of specific antibody to the specific antigen protein present on the exosome membrane (e.g. CD63). Magnet-based kits are commercially available for specific isolation of CD81, CD63, CD9 or EpCam-containing exosomes.

Using saccharide residues on the exosomal surface is also another approach in affinity methods [32]. This approach is easy to apply, however, due to the huge number of cells that contain

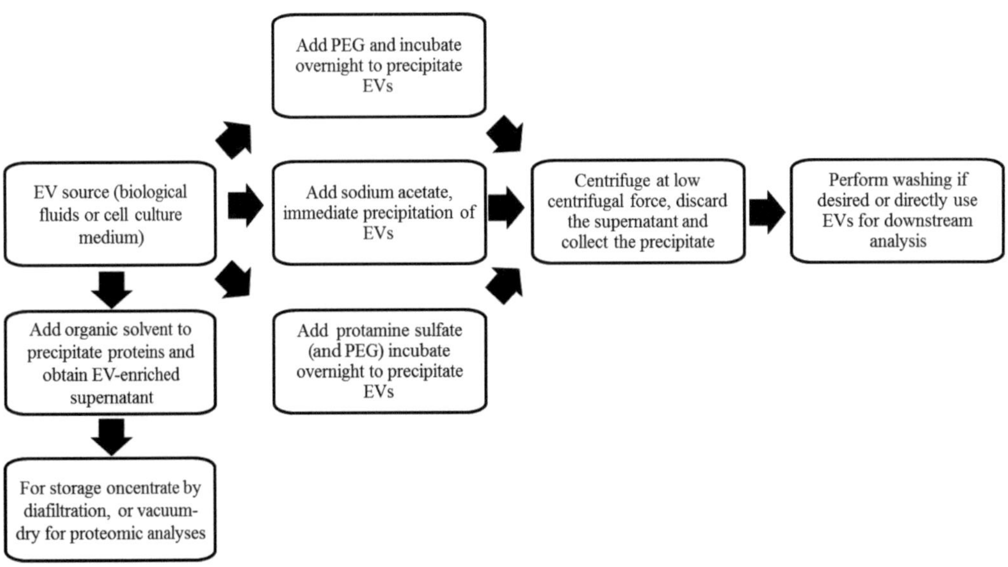

Figure 5. General steps followed during EV isolation by precipitation. One of the following methods of precipitation can be chosen by the researcher: protein organic solvent precipitation, polymer-driven precipitation, salting out with electrolyte solution or ionic precipitation by using cationic protamine. After an incubation period, the precipitate is collected by low-speed centrifugation.

mannose on their surface, the specificity of this affinity method is weak. Another affinity-based method relies on heparin affinity of EV. Based on previous observations that heparin blocks entry of EVs to recipient cells, a group of researchers hypothesized that heparin can bind directly to heparin sulphate proteoglycans on EVs' surface and can be used for their isolation [33]. Like in the case with saccharide affinity, the fact that many cell types contain heparin sulphate proteoglycans the specificity of this capturing method is weak too. Different steps needed in affinity-based approaches for EV isolation can be seen in **Figure 6**.

4.5. Commercial isolation kits

The increased research on exosomes for diagnostic and therapeutic applications has led to the development of commercially available isolation kits. Commercial kits for EV isolation involve precipitation of the proteins on the outer membrane of EVs along with contaminating proteins of non-EV origin. So, it is very important to determine the contaminating proteins before using their quantity for normalization of further experiments. Commercial kits for AV isolation include column-based isolation kits, immunocapture-based isolation kits and precipitation-based kits. **Table 2** summarizes the commercially available exosome isolation kits. Each of these kits is designed for isolating extracellular vesicles for various post-isolation applications, and can be found on the manufacturers' product lists.

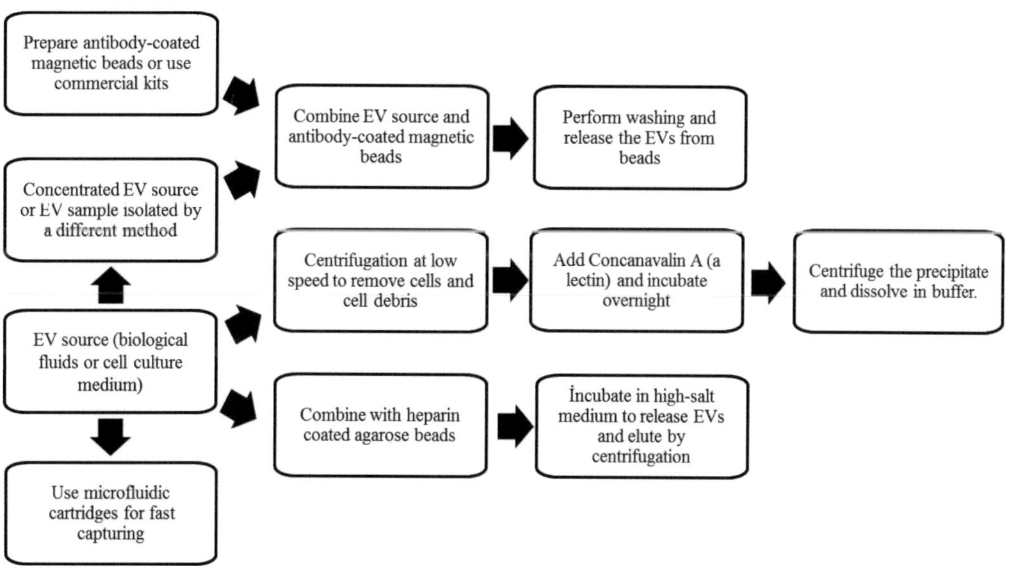

Figure 6. Main steps followed during different affinity-based EV isolation methods. Antibody affinity, lectin affinity or heparin affinity can be employed depending on specific properties of expected EVs. For antibody affinity, a concentrated source medium or EV isolate previously obtained by another method is combined and incubated with antibody coated beads or plates. Afterwards, the exosomes are washed and eluted. For lectin affinity isolation, a low-speed centrifugation is performed in order to eliminate intact cells and cell debris, and the medium is incubated in the presence of lectins. Then EVs, selectively bound to the lectins, are collected by centrifugation. For heparin affinity isolation, the EV source is combined with heparin-coated agarose beads and incubated. Later, EVs are released by adding concentrated salt solution and eluted by centrifugation. Very promising alternative is the use of microfluidic devices pre-coated with antibodies. This method ensures very fast capturing of specific EV subtypes.

Name of the commercial kit	Manufacturer	Principle
ExoCap™ exosome isolation kit	JRS Life Sciences GmbH Co.	İmmunocapture and magnetic separation
Exosome-Human CD81/CD63/CD9/ EpCAM isolation kits	Life Technologies Inc.	İmmunocapture and magnetic separation
Exo-spin™ exosome purification kit	Cell Guidance Systems Ltd.	Sedimentation and column filtration
qEV Size Exclusion Column	iZON Ltd.	Size exclusion chromatography
Invitrogen total exosome isolation kit	Life Technologies Inc.	Sedimentation
ExoQuick™ and ExoQuick-TC™ exosome isolation kits	System Biosciences	Sedimentation
ME™ exosome isolation kit	New England Peptide	Sedimentation
miRCURY™ exosome isolation kit	Exiquon Inc.	Sedimentation

Table 2. Commercially available kits for extracellular vesicle isolation.

When, the commercial ExoQuick exosome isolation kit was compared with classical ultracentrifugation, ExoQuick revealed ca. 19 times higher protein quantity in the isolated exosomal dispersion and is proven simpler and faster [34]. Yet no further experiments are performed to clarify if all the protein yields are truly of exosomal origin. Optiprep density gradient was successfully used for separation of exosomes, microvesicles, free proteins, non-exosome small vesicles and proteasome from the same cells [19].

5. Comparison of exosome isolation methods in diagnosis and treatment of cancer

Table 3 gives examples of studies on EV isolation methods and summarizes the major findings.

As previously mentioned, in order to be applicable for therapeutic purpose, EV product should have a clearly defined origin and well-characterized particles with homogeneous size distribution. Because different EV subtypes are generated by different biogenesis pathways and originate from distinct cellular parts, their molecular cargo differs significantly. Therefore, when EVs will be used for delivery of specific small RNA molecules generated in the donor cells, it is crucial to distinguish whether obtained EVs are microvesicles or exosomes. While for particular applications such as RNA delivery or drug delivery exosomes may be preferable, for other applications such as vaccination and surface antigen display microvesicles might be more relevant [40]. For diagnostic application, especially in proteomics analyses, free protein contaminants may lead to false-positive results. In so far as diagnosis is performed on body fluid samples, attention should be paid to numerous contamination factors like viruses, serum/plasma components, bacteria etc. Suitable method or combination of methods should be selected in order to eliminate all these factors that would affect final results.

Researchers should first consider the downstream application and then decide which method to use according to their advantages and disadvantages. These features of the methods mentioned in this chapter are summarized below.

http://dx.doi.org/10.5772/intechopen.69407

Source of EVs	Origin	Isolation method(s) used	Findings and outcomes
Cell culture media	CD14+ monocyte-derived dendritic cells from healthy donors	• Ultrafiltration → cushion ultracentrifugation • Filtration → centrifugation → cushion ultracentrifugation • Differential Centrifugation	Ultrafiltration followed by cushion ultracentrifugation has given a stable exosome yield with higher recovery, and regulatory compliance. The method of differential centrifugation produced highly variable results with less effective exosome yield [17]
Whole blood	Healthy donors	• Differential centrifugation • ExoQuick (Precipitation)	Two methods are compared with regard to how they affect the miRNA profile of the isolated exosomes. Comparable results were reported. ExoQuick is not recommended for obtaining exosomes intended for further biochemical and immunological studies [35]
Cell culture media/ biological fluids	NS	Differential centrifugation	Step-by-step description of the ultracentrifugation method is provided [36]
Cell culture media	LIM1863 colon cancer cell line	• Ultracentrifugation • Density gradient separation (OptiPrep) • Immunoaffinity capture	The least yield was achieved by ultracentrifugation, followed by OptiPrep, and the best was achieved by immunoaffinity capture. Ultracentrifugation was the faster method with only 2 hours required to complete. The immunoaffinity has considered the best method [18]
Cell culture media	U87 and 293T cancer cells and normal HUVE cells	• Heparin affinity separation • Ultracentrifugation • ExoQuick	Using the affinity of EVs for heparin, researchers succeeded to demonstrate a simple and effective method to isolate highly pure populations of EVs [33]
Cell culture media	K1735P melanoma cell line	• Ultracentrifugation • Salting-out procedure	Simple and cost-effective ion neutralization in acetate buffer media is described. Increased protein yield is observed in comparison to ultracentrifugation [25]
Cell culture media	Huh-7 liver cancer cell line	• Ultracentrifugation • ExoQuick (Precipitation)	ExoQuick revealed higher protein quantity in the isolated exosomal dispersion, and has been proven simpler and faster [34]. Yet, it still remains to be clarified if the proteins are not of extraneous origin
Cell culture media	MDA231 breast cancer cell line	• Sequential filtration • Differential ultracentrifugation	Vesicles with much greater poly-dispersity are obtained with the sequential filtration method. Exosomal preparations with very high purity are obtained [22]
Body fluids	Platelet concentrate	• Size exclusion chromatography	Efficient, single step, rapid and cost-effective EV isolation method is described [12]
Cell culture media	D3 murine embryonic stem cell line	• Differential ultracentrifugation; • Centrifugal extrusion of whole cells to produce exosome-mimetic vesicles	Based on the protein and RNA amount in obtained EVs whole cell-extrusion method has given nearly 250 times higher vesicle yield than simple exosome isolation [37]. Also, similar results were obtained with in vitro delivery studies

Source of EVs	Origin	Isolation method(s) used	Findings and outcomes
Cell culture media	D3 murine embryonic stem cell line	• Differential centrifugation; • Microfluidics-mediated extrusion of whole cells to produce exosome-mimetic vesicles	Researchers compared the two methods for production of cell-derived vesicles but no comparison of the protein and vesicle yield vas made [38]. Similar results were observed with EVs isolated with both methods in *in vitro* delivery studies
Cell culture media	BT-474 breast cancer cell line	• Differential ultracentrifugation • ExoSpin Exosome Purification Kit • Invitrogen Total Exosome Purification Kit • PureExo Exosome Isolation Kit	All four methods are considered non-specific for exosome isolation because of the presence of large particles [39].
Cell culture media	Monocyte-derived dendritic cells, HEK293T, RPE-1, HeLa-CIITA, MDA-MB-231, SHIN, IGROV-1, OV2008	• Differential ultracentrifugation • Optiprep/Iodixanol gradient ultracentrifugation • Sucrose gradient ultracentrifugation • Immunoaffinity capture	Subtypes of EVs were isolated by combining different methods such as ultracentrifugation and iodixanol gradient. Subgroups of small non exosomal vesicles, not carrying the exosomal markers were described [19]

Table 3. Studies dealing with EV isolation and major findings thereof.

5.1. Centrifugation-based methods

Advantages

- these methods are recognized as gold standard for isolation of extracellular vesicles
- as the most commonly used method, ultracentrifugation is acceptable for isolating EVs for many application purposes
- well-established protocols and troubleshooting are available
- ultracentrifugation can be used in combination with other techniques in order to provide better resolution of microvesicles and exosomes
- differential ultracentrifugation is able to discriminate between exosomes, small non-exosome vesicles and microvesicles owing to their different buoyant density

Disadvantages

- the yield of EVs is highly varying in different setups
- requirement for expensive instrumentation and consumables

- disposable consumables like ultracentrifuge tubes meaning
- information about the rotor type and geometry, applied g-force, solution viscosity and salinity should all be considered in order to achieve reproducible results
- the procedure of ultracentrifugation is very time laborious and requires substantial amount of hands-on work. The density gradient ultracentrifugation takes even more time with extra purification steps from start to finish
- in differential ultracentrifugation, not only exosomes are being collected at the end of the isolation. Therefore, for both diagnostic and therapeutic applications, isolates should be purified from contaminating proteins and other EV subtypes in order to avoid

5.2. Size exclusion chromatography

Advantages

- exosomes are isolated in a single step
- short operation time
- efficient elimination of contaminating proteins
- efficient separation of EV subtypes (provided that the sample loading volume is not too large)
- high purity of EV isolates
- no extra compounds are added in order to perform the isolation

Disadvantages

- samples are collected as a large number of fractions
- need to characterize each fraction in order to ensure presence of EVs and proteins
- requirement for aseptic working conditions in order to prevent microbial contamination
- exosomes and small non-exosome vesicles cannot be separated
- large sample loading volume may lead to inefficient separation

5.3. Filtration-based isolation

Advantages

- effective separation of exosomes and microvesicles
- simple and short operation
- efficient elimination of contaminating proteins
- efficient separation of EV subtypes (exosomes and microvesicles)
- high purity of EV isolates

- the method is able to handle large-volume sample
- no extra compounds are added in order to perform the isolation
- suitable for development of microfluidic isolation setups

Disadvantages

- the method cannot be applied on small-volume samples
- exosomes and small non-exosome vesicles cannot be discriminated
- possibility of occlusion of membranes during operation
- membranes should be carefully regenerated or discarded after use

5.4. Precipitation-based isolation

Advantages

- ability to precipitate virtually all EVs in the biological sample
- very high yield
- versatility to perform isolation in different precipitation protocols
- fast and easy application
- protein solvent precipitation method may enhance diagnostic strength of exosomes and ensure contaminant-free isolates for therapeutic applications

Disadvantages

- need to remove the precipitating polymer or salt for downstream applications
- production of highly heterogeneous and protein-contaminated EV mixture
- need for extra purification steps

5.5. Affinity-based methods

Advantages

- provides specific isolation of individual EV subpopulations
- high-purity EV production
- suitable for development of microfluidic isolation setups

Disadvantages

- requirement of specific antibodies and targeting ligands
- need of solid knowledge about EVs' structure
- possibility of functionality loss after detachment from antibodies
- not suitable for high-volume samples

6. Conclusion

Exosomes are gaining continuously increasing interest in biological, medical and pharmaceutical research fields. Treatment and diagnosis of cancer are two particularly promising applications of exosomes. Isolation methods for exosomes are being advanced with the time and new modifications to available methods are being introduced. According to the available literature, there is still no method that is free of shortages. For both applications, scientists should consider carefully the advantages and disadvantages of available methods. It is obvious from published methods that immunoaffinity isolation promises specific capture of exosomes from biological fluids, taking advantage of their membrane structures. Therefore, in cases where exosomes will be subject of investigation for diagnosis of cancer, immunoaffinity may provide isolation of exosomes in the most sensitive and specific manner among all methods. By hyphenation of affinity methods to microfluidics field, even faster isolation, detection and analysis of exosomes can be achieved. The question of 'which method is the best?' currently remains unanswered for therapeutic applications of exosomes. Regulatory requirements for a standardized clinical grade exosome isolation method are yet to be established. Nevertheless, size exclusion chromatography and ultrafiltration methods which do not require incorporation of extra compounds to facilitate the isolation provide exosome isolates with high purity. For cancer therapy, these two methods may be considered optimal.

Author details

Mustafa Kotmakçı[1]* and Gülşah Erel Akbaba[2]

*Address all correspondence to: mustafa.kotmakci@ege.edu.tr

1 Department of Pharmaceutical Biotechnology, Faculty of Pharmacy, Ege University, Izmir, Turkey

2 Department of Pharmaceutical Biotechnology, Faculty of Pharmacy, Izmir Katip Çelebi University, Izmir, Turkey

References

[1] Vader P, Mol EA, Pasterkamp G, Schiffelers RM. Extracellular vesicles for drug delivery. Adv Drug Deliv Rev. 2016;**106**:148-56

[2] Vlassov A V., Magdaleno S, Setterquist R, Conrad R. Exosomes: Current knowledge of their composition, biological functions, and diagnostic and therapeutic potentials. Biochim Biophys Acta - Gen Subj. 2012;**1820**(7):940-8

[3] Ji H, Chen M, Greening DW, He W, Rai A, Zhang W, et al. Deep sequencing of RNA from three different extracellular vesicle (EV) subtypes released from the human LIM1863 colon cancer cell line uncovers distinct miRNA-enrichment signatures. PLoS One. 2014;**9**(10):e110314

[4] Webber J, Clayton A. How pure are your vesicles? J Extracell vesicles. 2013;**2**:19861

[5] Lobb RJ, Becker M, Wen Wen S, Wong CSF, Wiegmans AP, Leimgruber A, et al. Optimized exosome isolation protocol for cell culture supernatant and human plasma. J Extracell Vesicles. 2015;**4**:27031

[6] JJin Y, Chen K, Wang Z, Wang Y, Liu J, Lin L, et al. DNA in serum extracellular vesicles is stable under different storage conditions. BMC Cancer. 2016;**16**:753

[7] Witwer KW, Buzás EI, Bemis LT, Bora A, Lässer C, Lötvall J, et al. Standardization of sample collection, isolation and analysis methods in extracellular vesicle research. J Extracell Vesicles. 2013;**2**:20360

[8] Tataruch-Weinert D, Musante L, Kretz O, Holthofer H. Urinary extracellular vesicles for RNA extraction: optimization of a protocol devoid of prokaryote contamination. J Extracell Vesicles. 2016;**5**:30281

[9] Lener T, Gimona M, Aigner L, Börger V, Buzas E, Camussi G, et al. Applying extracellular vesicles based therapeutics in clinical trials - an ISEV position paper. J Extracell Vesicles. 2015;**4**:30087

[10] Shin H, Han C, Labuz JM, Kim J, Kim J, Cho S, et al. High-yield isolation of extracellular vesicles using aqueous two-phase system. Sci Rep. 2015;14;**5**:13103

[11] Baranyai T, Herczeg K, Onódi Z, Voszka I, Módos K, Marton N, et al. Isolation of Exosomes from Blood Plasma: Qualitative and Quantitative Comparison of Ultracentrifugation and Size Exclusion Chromatography Methods. PLoS One. 2015;**10**(12):e0145686

[12] Böing AN, van der Pol E, Grootemaat AE, Coumans FAW, Sturk A, Nieuwland R. Single-step isolation of extracellular vesicles by size-exclusion chromatography. J Extracell Vesicles. 2014;**3**:23430

[13] Nordin JZ, Lee Y, Vader P, Mäger I, Johansson HJ, Heusermann W, et al. Ultrafiltration with size-exclusion liquid chromatography for high yield isolation of extracellular vesicles preserving intact biophysical and functional properties. Nanomedicine: Nanotechnology, Biology and Medicine. 2015;**11**(4):879-883

[14] Chiou N-T, Ansel KM. Improved exosome isolation by sucrose gradient fractionation of ultracentrifuged crude exosome pellets [Internet]. Protocol Exchange. 2016 [cited 2017 Jan]. Available from: http://www.nature.com/protocolexchange/protocols/5035

[15] Taylor DD, Shah S. Methods of isolating extracellular vesicles impact down-stream analyses of their cargoes. Methods. 2015;**87**:3-10

[16] Johnstone RM, Adam M, Hammond JR, Orr L, Turbide C. Vesicle formation during reticulocyte maturation. Association of plasma membrane activities with released vesicles (exosomes). J Biol Chem. 1987;**262**(19):9412-20

[17] Lamparski HG, Metha-Damani A, Yao J-Y, Patel S, Hsu D-H, Ruegg C, et al. Production and characterization of clinical grade exosomes derived from dendritic cells. J Immunol Methods. 2002;**270**(2):211-26

[18] Tauro BJ, Greening DW, Mathias R a, Ji H, Mathivanan S, Scott AM, et al. Comparison of ultracentrifugation, density gradient separation, and immunoaffinity capture methods for isolating human colon cancer cell line LIM1863-derived exosomes. Methods. 2012;**56**(2):293-304

[19] Kowal J, Arras G, Colombo M, Jouve M, Morath JP, Primdal-Bengtson B, et al. Proteomic comparison defines novel markers to characterize heterogeneous populations of extracellular vesicle subtypes. Proc Natl Acad Sci U S A. 2016;**113**(8):E968-77

[20] Van Deun J, Mestdagh P, Sormunen R, Cocquyt V, Vermaelen K, Vandesompele J, et al. The impact of disparate isolation methods for extracellular vesicles on downstream RNA profiling. J Extracell Vesicles. 2014;**3**:24858

[21] Musante L, Tataruch DE, Holthofer H. Use and isolation of urinary exosomes as biomarkers for diabetic nephropathy. Front Endocrinol (Lausanne). 2014;**5**:1-12

[22] Heinemann ML, Ilmer M, Silva LP, Hawke DH, Recio A, Vorontsova MA, et al. Benchtop isolation and characterization of functional exosomes by sequential filtration. J Chromatogr A. 2014;**1371**:125-35

[23] Deregibus MC, Figliolini F, D'Antico S, Manzini PM, Pasquino C, De Lena M, et al. Charge-based precipitation of extracellular vesicles. Int J Mol Med. 2016;**38**(5):1359-66

[24] Weng Y, Sui Z, Shan Y, Hu Y, Chen Y, Zhang L, et al. Effective isolation of exosomes with polyethylene glycol from cell culture supernatant for in-depth proteome profiling. Analyst. 2016;**141**(15):4640-6

[25] Brownlee Z, Lynn KD, Thorpe PE, Schroit AJ. A novel "salting-out" procedure for the isolation of tumor-derived exosomes. J Immunol Methods. 2014;**407**:120-6

[26] Ban J-J, Lee M, Im W, Kim M. Low pH increases the yield of exosome isolation. Biochem Biophys Res Commun. 2015;**461**(1):76-79

[27] Gallart-Palau X, Serra A, Wong ASW, Sandin S, Lai MKP, Chen CP, et al. Extracellular vesicles are rapidly purified from human plasma by PRotein Organic Solvent PRecipitation (PROSPR). Sci Rep. 2015;**5**:14664

[28] Greening DW, Xu R, Ji H, Tauro BJ, Simpson RJ. A Protocol for Exosome Isolation and Characterization: Evaluation of Ultracentrifugation, Density-Gradient Separation, and Immunoaffinity Capture Methods. Methods in Molecular Biology. 2015;**1295**:179-209

[29] Chen C, Skog J, Hsu C-H, Lessard RT, Balaj L, Wurdinger T, et al. Microfluidic isolation and transcriptome analysis of serum microvesicles. Lab Chip. 2010;**10**(4):505-11

[30] Im H, Shao H, Park Y Il, Peterson VM, Castro CM, Weissleder R, et al. Label-free detection and molecular profiling of exosomes with a nano-plasmonic sensor. Nat Biotechnol. 2014;**32**(5):490-5

[31] Kanwar SS, Dunlay CJ, Simeone DM, Nagrath S. Microfluidic device (ExoChip) for on-chip isolation, quantification and characterization of circulating exosomes. Lab Chip. 2014;**14**(11):1891

[32] Samsonov R, Shtam T, Burdakov V, Glotov A, Tsyrlina E, Berstein L, et al. Lectin-induced agglutination method of urinary exosomes isolation followed by mi-RNA analysis: Application for prostate cancer diagnostic. Prostate. 2016;**76**(1):68-79

[33] Balaj L, Atai NA, Chen W, Mu D, Tannous BA, Breakefield XO, et al. Heparin affinity purification of extracellular vesicles. Sci Rep. 2015;**5**:10266

[34] Zhu L, Qu X-H, Sun Y-L, Qian Y-M, Zhao X-H. Novel method for extracting exosomes of hepatocellular carcinoma cells. World J Gastroenterol. 2014;**20**(21):6651-7

[35] Rekker K, Saare M, Roost AM, Kubo A-L, Zarovni N, Chiesi A, et al. Comparison of serum exosome isolation methods for microRNA profiling. Clin Biochem. 2014;**47**(1-2):135-8

[36] Lässer C, Eldh M, Lötvall J. Isolation and characterization of RNA-containing exosomes. J Vis Exp. 2012;(59):e3037

[37] Jo W, Kim J, Yoon J, Jeong D, Cho S, Jeong H, et al. Large-scale generation of cell-derived nanovesicles. Nanoscale. 2014;**6**(20):12056-64

[38] Jo W, Jeong D, Kim J, Cho S, Jang SC, Han C, et al. Microfluidic fabrication of cell-derived nanovesicles as endogenous RNA carriers. Lab Chip. 2014;**14**(7):1261-9

[39] Lane RE, Korbie D, Anderson W, Vaidyanathan R, Trau M. Analysis of exosome purification methods using a model liposome system and tunable-resistive pulse sensing. Sci Rep. 2015;**5**:7639

[40] Sedlik C, Vigneron J, Torrieri-Dramard L, Pitoiset F, Denizeau J, Chesneau C, et al. Different immunogenicity but similar antitumor efficacy of two DNA vaccines coding for an antigen secreted in different membrane vesicle-associated forms. J Extracell Vesicles. 2014;**3**(1):24646